ALLE ZEIT WACH
SJ
1842

Georg Riccabona

Thyroid Cancer

Its Epidemiology
Clinical Features, and Treatment

With 44 Figures and 48 Tables

Springer-Verlag Berlin Heidelberg New York
London Paris Tokyo

Professor Dr. Georg Riccabona
Universitätsklinik für Nuklearmedizin
Anichstraße 35
A-6020 Innsbruck

ISBN-13:978-3-642-71212-8 e-ISBN-13:978-3-642-71210-4
DOI: 10.1007/978-3-642-71210-4

Library of Congress Cataloging in Publication Data
Riccabona, G. (Georg) Thyroid cancer. Includes bibliographies and index. 1. Thyroid gland–Cancer. I. Title. [DNLM: 1. Thyroid Neoplasms. WK 270 R491t]
RC280.T6R53 1987 616.99'444 87-13131 ISBN-13:978-3-642-71212-8 (U.S.)

Softcover reprint of the hardcover 1st edition 1987

2127/3145-543210

To my dear wife Fee in gratitude
for her love and patience

Preface

The idea to publish a "compendium" on Thyroid Cancer came to me a few years ago, when I noticed the increasing discrepancies in the medical community concerning classification of thyroid neoplasms, management of thyroid cancer patients and prognosis of the disease. With all the discussions about this rare, but peculiar disease it is finally the patient with such a lesion, who has to bear the consequences of therapeutic decisions. The question "When is malignant goiter malignant?" (Ward 1949) still remains open. Local differences in the clinical course and the prognosis of thyroid malignancies persist and can influence the therapeutic approach. I am aware of the fact, that thyroid cancer – in it's morphology, etiology, clinical picture and therapy – is indeed not one disease but a group of partly different nosological entities.

This booklet should therefore not be considered as a fundamental publication covering the subject "in extenso". It should, however, be applied as an outline, how the surgeon or physician in charge should proceed in patients with the suspicion of thyroid malignancy, taking into account the fascinating data acquired during recent years in the broad spectrum of basic sciences, such as immunohistochemistry, pathophysiology, etiological considerations etc.

This publication could never have been presented without the valuable help of all my collaborators (Dr. Heiko Fill, Dr. Anton Fink, Dr. Elisabeth Hilty, Dr. Michael Oberladstätter, Dr. Wolfgang Zechmann) and without the secretarial skills of Mrs. Gisela Öhlzelt. Furthermore I would like to acknowledge the invaluable roles of my teachers – the late Prof. Dr. Paul Huber and Prof. John B. Stanbury – who have deeply influenced my scientific and clinical approach to thyroid disease in general. I also would like to acknowledge the competent advice of Prof. Ferdinand Hofstädter and Dr. Kurt Schmid from out Pathology Department and especially the comments of Dr. Christopher Marsh from the Language School of our University concerning a proper expression in English. Finally I thank Dr. J. Wieczorek of Springer-Editions for his advice and cooperation during the preparation of this manuscript.

Innsbruck, 1987 G. Riccabona

Table of Contents

A General Aspects and Basic Sciences

B Clinical Picture, Diagnosis, Therapy and Follow-up

A
General Aspects and Basic Sciences

Introduction and Historical Review

We do not know exactly when and how thyroid malignancy was first recognized as a well defined disease. During the middle ages it may well have been a part of the "tumidum guttur"-syndrome (= neck tumor), which also included tuberculosis of cervical lymph nodes and a variety of other diseases (Merke 1971). In old Egypt, however, and then in the famous Medical School of Salerno surgical treatment of such neck tumors was already known (Major 1954; Denies et al. 1958). On the other hand some therapeutic nihilism regarding such lesions was widespread and the afflicted patients were often treated with magic or other non-scientific methods ("Le Roy te touche, Dieu te guerit = The king touches you and the Lord will heal") (Merke 1971). To my knowledge it was J. Beck (1833) who published the first documented case of malignant goiter (Fig. 1). By the time when Kocher made thyroid surgery really feasible, he had already described thyroid cancer and it's treatment (Kocher 1924). In 1925 Breitner noted (Breitner 1925), however, that thyroid malignancies in general were killing patients within 1 year and even in 1938 (Urban 1938) a cure of thyroid cancer was considered as a "glücklicher Zufall" (= lucky chance). Dur-

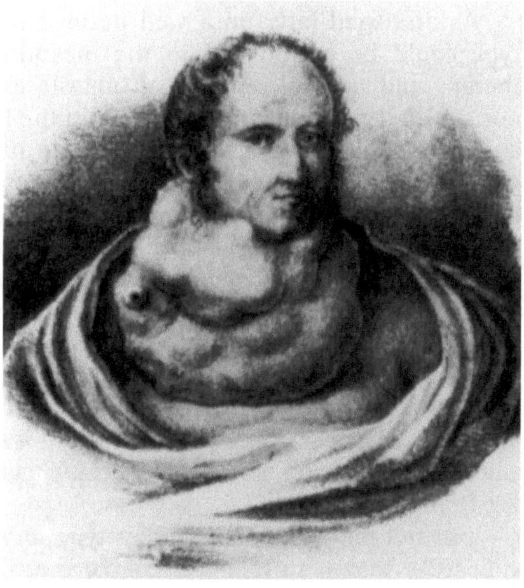

Fig. 1. Probably oldest picture of thyroid cancer patient (Beck J. „Über den Kropf, ein Beitrag zur Pathologie und Therapie desselben", Freiburg i. Br. 1833)

ing the first half of our century pathologists studied thyroid cancer in detail and were frequently puzzled by the different histological patterns of these tumors (Wegelin 1926): They tried to classify thyroid cancer in detail and sometimes with odd nomenclatures: "Metastasizing Adenoma", "wuchernde" (= proliferating) Struma Langhans and other terms were applied and cervical lymphnode metastases of thyroid cancer were frequently classified as "aberrant thyroid tissue" (Lahey; Ficarra 1946). Only the introduction of radioiodine in diagnosis and therapy provided a break-through in the understanding, diagnosis and therapy of this disease (Hamilton; Soley 1943). Even as from one year to another further informations become available regarding aetiology, pathology and the clinical management of thyroid malignancies it seems more evident than ever, that thyroid cancer is indeed a complex of different tumor types with their well defined morphological, clinical and prognostic peculiarities.

As thyroid cancer is no common disease scientific evaluation has often been impaired by small case series, reports on the subject were frequently case studies. Nevertheless 2 opposite trends in the management of thyroid cancer became obvious in the last 40 years and – to some extent – they exist even now. An impressive clinical description of thyroid cancer was presented also by Albrecht in 1893 (Albrecht 1893). Actually we have to consider:

1. Radical and/or ultraradical therapeutic strategy
Total thyroidectomy, wide use of sternotomy, "prophylactic" radical neck dissection were proposed by several authors (Dargent 1948; Clark et al. 1969) together with routine postoperative radiotherapy (Pemberton 1939) and ^{131}I-therapy.
2. Other well established teams suggested only *limited surgical procedures sometimes unilaterally together with thyroid hormone therapy* (Becker et al. 1984; Thomas 1957). They did not include ^{131}I or percutaneous irradiation in their primary therapeutic programs.

As discussed later on a well defined therapeutic approach for each tumor type could be established in the meantime, which – together with chemotherapy and surgical removal of metastases – has helped to improve the prognosis of thyroid cancer significantly in the last 2 decades. Thyroid cancer is not a disease which always shows up due to its superficial location in early tumor stages and is sometimes only detected when distant metastases are present. Nuclear medicine, sonography, and fine needle biopsy helped very much – sometimes together with CT-scanning and nuclear magnetic resonance imaging (NMRI) – to estabilish a correct diagnosis in due time for appropriate therapy.

The possibility to study thyroid cancer in cell cultures (Andreoli et al. 1981) with all the techniques of modern biosciences is constantly providing us with new knowledge on this disease but although there are maybe more answers, a lot of new questions arise. Does C-cell carcinoma really grow exclusively from branchiogenic, parafollicular cells? Will well-differentiated thyroid adeno-carcinomas at a given time change into anaplastic tumors (Huber; Riccabona 1967) and if so, why?

I cannot remember one cancer type to which – in contrast to it's frequency and death rate – so many scientific meetings were dedicated in recent years.

This shows that obviously thyroid cancer can – to a certain degree – serve as a practical tumor model in which many variables can easily be studied and from which important therapeutic decisions can be derived. Under these circumstances it is obvious that the information given in the following chapters may have a short "half-life". On the other hand I would like to quote from a relevant paper a very fitting statement made in the first decades of our century (Breitner 1925): "If the neoplasm is removed when it is restricted to the thyroid gland and no metastases are present a cure can be achieved which may last for decades" and "It is important to know that a solitary metastasis of thyroid carcinoma is no fatal verdict for the patient: Removal of the metastasis and the primary lesion can provide a long-term cure". Obviously therefore older and more recent experiences should be kept in mind when we talk about thyroid cancer and when we would like to apply our knowledge to our patients.

The data presented in the following pages are essentially an interpretation of a well-documented series of 1493 thyroid cancer patients seen in our service from 1956–1984, mostly with long-term follow-up for up to 25 years. Of course our data are compared with informations from the international literature to exclude any bias and to provide a comprehensive presentation of the subject. As – since many years – the Nuclear Medicine Service of our University is the largest Center for high dose ^{131}I-therapy in Austria we have to admit, however, that epidemiological data could not be considered as representative for patients from outside of the province of Tyrol to some extent, especially as also patients from southern Germany and northern Italy were admitted to our service. We took great care to restrict epidemiological data only to patients from the Tyrol province. Also it should be mentioned that due to a high incidence of endemic goiter iodized salt goiter prophylaxis was introduced legally in Austria in 1963 (Österr. BGBl., 1963) and that this program obviously modified the pattern of thyroid cancer as described later on. Actually the normal table salt in Austria is iodized by law at a level of 1:100000, providing an average I-urine excretion of ~65 mcg/g creatinine (Riccabona 1972). In all the discussions in the following chapters one should never forget, that untreated or inadequately treated thyroid cancer is a disease which kills patients often only after terrible suffering: asphyxia, dysphagia, severe pain due to nerve irritation, immobility due to bone metastases etc. are all symptoms, which make these patients really "sick" and every effort to avoid the sequelae of thyroid cancer should therefore be made. Such efforts, however, can only be efficient when we understand the specific manifestations and behaviour patterns of thyroid malignancy. As outlined later on, it will be one goal of this publication to define risk groups for thyroid cancer, to establish more detailed high risk groups in the context of thyroid malignancies and to discuss the reasons for these various options as well as proposals for adequate therapy. This should also help to promote a world-wide, well coordinated study of the problem. Between resignation and highly active treatment we should define our approach to each individual case on the basis of ample knowledge, careful decision and personal responsibility.

Epidemiology

1 General Aspects

It is a pity that information on the epidemiology of thyroid cancer is so inadequate. I suggested years ago that a more profound and sweeping investigation should be carried out by the WHO regarding the subject, but obviously no reliable data can be presented today, as epidemiological studies of such a relatively rare disease in developing countries – which make up about 70% of the world population by now – can scarcely be realized. Therefore many, potentially valuable data on incidence and classification of thyroid cancer in different age groups and in males or females are missing in this presentation. One general trend can be observed however (Table 1): There is a definite prevalence of thyroid cancer in females as compared to males, while the sex ratio of thyroid diseases overall is even higher for females and the age distribution shows peaks above the 4th decade. It should be noted that – in contrast to many other solid tumors – children and adolescents can also be afflicted by the disease in significant numbers. An unanswered question is the discrepancy between the high incidence of thyroid cancer in routine autopsy series in contrast to the clinical incidence of malignant goiter and even more to the death rate due to thyroid malignancies (Table 2). It is certainly impossible to classify histologically all the thyroid cancers detected in routine autopsy series as malignant tumors. On the other hand we know (Fukunaga, Lockett 1971) that "latent" thyroid carcinoma can – after many years – become a clinically impressive disease. No adequate definition exists at present regarding the prospective outcome of histologically malignant thyroid lesions in individual cases. We do know, however, the death rates due to thyroid cancer (Table 3) and from these data it becomes obvious, that the prognosis of thyroid cancer is – in general – worse in endemic goiter countries than in goiter-free areas. The exception to

Table 1. Age and sex distribution of thyroid cancer

Age and incidence (own material) [yrs]		Sex ratio males/females (own material)
<20	4%	
21 – 40	20%	
41 – 60	35%	1:2.63
>60	41%	

Table 2. Incidence of thyroid cancer in routine autopsy series, as clinically relevant cases and death rate due to thyroid cancer

	Source	Country	Incidence
Autopsy material	Williams 1983	USA, Japan	>20%
	Sasaki et al. 1976	Japan	8%
	Sampson et al. 1974	USA	6%
Clinical cases	Mustacchi Cutler 1957	USA	2.9/100000/year
	Steinitz 1974	Israel	5/100000/year
	Hedinger 1969	Colombia, Hawaii	10/100000/year
	Riccabona 1984	Austria	3.8/100000/year
Death rates	Riccabona 1985	Austria 1952	1.62/100000/year
(Age adjusted)		Austria 1983	1.07/100000/year
	Kurihara et al. 1984	Switzerland 1952	1.79/100000/year
		Switzerland 1979	0.87/100000/year
		USA 1979	0.31/100000/year
		Israel 1952	0.89/100000/year
		UK 1963	0.66/100000/year

Table 3. Death rates of thyroid cancer with special regard to endemic goiter

	Source	Country	Death rates	Goiter prevalence
Endemic	Riccabona 1980	Austria	1.62/100.000/year	35%
goiter areas	Stanbury, Hetzel 1980	Colombia	?	53%
	Kurihara 1984	Yugoslavia	1.9/100000/year	~28%
		Finland	1.5/100000/year	22%
		Israel	1.01/100000/year	~30%
Only	Kurihara 1984	USA	0.3/100000/year	<10%
sporadic	Riccabona 1980	UK	0.45/100.000/year	<10%
goiter	Stanbury, Hetzel 1980	Japan	0.40/100000/year	<10%
Mixed areas	Riccabona 1980	Chile	0.48/100000/year?	~11–30%
	Oberdisse et al. 1980	FRG	0.52/100000/year	16.5%
		Switzerland	0.8/100000/year	~25%

this rule is the fact, that in some developing countries without endemic goiter patients seek medical therapy only in advanced stages of the disease (El Haddad 1984). Is histopathology the ultimate answer for the biological behaviour of thyroid tumors? Can we define the incidence of thyroid cancer and it's epidemiology on the basis of microscopic pictures or rather on the basis of clinical experience? Should surgery be performed as a prophylactic measure in nodular goiters to inhibit malignant developments in such thyroid glands? For the last question there is an answer: 15% of thyroid cancers grow after initial surgery for benign nodular goiter (Huber, Riccabona 1969). Therefore "prophylactic surgery" of thyroid nodules does not seem justified. Whether future studies on serum thyroglobulin and possibly thyroid growth stimulating immunoglobulins can provide additional information on the high incidence of thyroid malignancies in recurrent goiters remains a task for future research.

In the chapter on aetiology another fascinating aspect of the epidemiology of thyroid cancer will be discussed in detail, it should briefly be mentioned already here: ionizing radiation on neck and upper chest – especially when applied during childhood – can induce thyroid cancer with a latent period of 10–20 years (Hempelmann et al. 1975). Whether the relatively high incidence of thyroid malignancy reported from Japan and Hawaii can generally be interpreted as late effects of atomic bomb-explosions in the Pacific Ocean area cannot be certified at present. The oncogenic effects of ionizing radiation in the thyroid will only be understood when precise epidemiological data are also obtained from regions with high natural radiation levels such as the highlands of Tibet in China, of Peru, Bolivia and of other regions in the world where natural radioactivity is elevated due to radioactive materials in the soil and in rocks (e.g. Kerala/India, southern Brazil).

A further epidemiological parameter is the incidence of thyroid cancer in single thyroid nodules in a young population (Oberdisse et al. 1980). Here – as discussed later on – a difference exists between data from endemic goiter areas and goiter-free regions. The probability of malignant thyroid disease in such lesions is quite high in goiter free zones while it is low in endemic goiter countries (Table 4). When such nodules are studied by isotope scanning and when they show up as "cold" nodules the probability of thyroid cancer becomes even higher, although different data are reported from endemic goiter regions and

Table 4. Incidence of thyroid cancer in single nodules in surgical series

Country	Source	Incidence
Austria	Keminger et al. 1975 (Vienna)	2.55%
FRG	Oberdisse et al. 1980	2.5%
India	Ram 1963	21.6%
USA	Cope et al. 1949 (Boston)	19.0%
	Crabtree, Hunter 1953 (Ann Arbor)	24.3%
	Lahey, Hare 1951 (Boston)	10.04%
	Hurxthal, Heinemann 1958 (Boston)	6.6%

Table 5. Incidence of thyroid cancer in cold nodules in endemic and sporadic goiter (surgical series)

Country	Goiter prevalence	Incidence	Source
Austria	35%	3.5%	Riccabona 1983
FRG	16.5%	~10.5%	Oberdisse et al. 1980
Greece	~20%	12.4%	Oberdisse et al. 1980
Sudan	~35%	1.5%	Oberdisse et al. 1980, Hetzel, Stanbury 1980
Switzerland	25%	22% [a]	Oberdisse et al. 1980
United Kingdom	<10%	11.4%	Oberdisse et al. 1980
USA	<10%	20.5%	Oberdisse et al. 1980

[a] Highly elected material!

goiter free areas (Riccabona 1980). In a period in which many classical endemic goiter countries have started some form of iodine prophylaxis (Ladurner et al. 1979), doctors should be aware of these facts, as with decreasing goiter incidence in a population the probability of thyroid malignancy increases in single cold nodules – especially in younger people (Galvan 1983). As the last lines show that endemic goiter can influence considerably the pattern and epidemiological criteria of thyroid cancer the following chapter will therefore be dedicated to discuss these relations in detail.

2 Correlation of Thyroid Cancer with Endemic Goiter

As mentioned previously, death rates due to thyroid cancer are high in endemic goiter countries and several classical authors (De Quervain 1941) felt, that thyroid cancer was more frequent in areas afflicted by endemic goiter than in goiter free regions. Recent data, however, show (Table 6) that the incidence of thyroid malignancy can also be high in areas without endemic goiter and adequate iodine supply (Hakama 1969). It was even suggested, that high iodine intake could induce the growth of papillary thyroid carcinoma (Williams et al. 1977). Obviously, therefore, no correlation between the incidence of thyroid cancer and endemic goiter due to iodine deficiency can be established on the basis of actual data (Stanbury, Hetzel 1980). On the other hand it is certain,

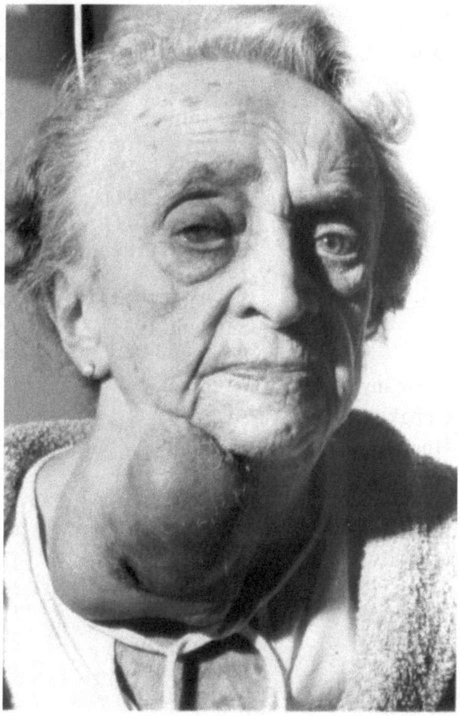

Fig. 2. Patient N. R., fem. 78 yrs., goiter since several decades, rapid growth with exulceration and spontaneous vocal chord paralysis since 6 months. Poorly differentiated follicular thyroid carcinoma

Table 6. Incidence of thyroid cancer in endemic goiter areas and goiter-free countries (+ sex ratios)

Country	Area	Incidence/ 100000/year	Females/ males	Source
Australia	NSW	1.6	2.55	Kurihara et al. 1984
	Urban	1.5	2.45	
	Rural	1.5	3.41	
	South	2.8	2.4	
	Average	1.85	2.7	
Austria	Tyrol 1980	1.65	1.6	Stanbury, Hetzel 1980
	Overall 1984	3.8	2.4	Fasching 1984
Belgium	Liège	2.2	?	Oberdisse et al. 1980
Brazil	São Paulo	2.7	2.4	Kurihara et al. 1984
Canada	Alberta	2.45	2.77	Kurihara et al. 1984
	Brit. Col.	2.35	2.35	
	Manitoba	2.80	2.30	
	Mar. Provs	2.10	3.2	
	Newfoundland	2.6	3.3	
	NWT & Yukon	1.50	> 3.0	
	Ontario	2.15	2.6	
	Quebec	1.18	2.3	
	Saskatchewan	3.3	2.5	
	Average	2.27	> 2.68	
5 provinces 1980	Average	1.75	2.9	Stanbury, Hetzel 1980
Chile	Average	1.45	2.2	Stanbury, Hetzel 1980
China	Shanghai	5.6	2.55	Kurihara et al. 1984
Colombia	Cali	3.75	4.15	Kurihara et al. 1984
ČSSR	Average	1.3	2.25	Kurihara et al. 1984
Cuba	Average	1.8	3.20	Kurihara et al. 1984
Denmark	Average	1.25	1.66	Kurihara et al. 1984
Finland	Average	2.75	2.35	Kurihara et al. 1984
France	Bas rhin	1.90	2.18	Kurihara et al. 1984
	Doubs	1.75	3.40	
	Average	1.82	2.79	
Germany, FRG	Hamburg 1974	3.14	1.02	Oberdisse et al. 1980
	Hamburg 1983	1.25	2.12	Kurihara et al. 1984
	Baden-Württemberg 1974	3.15	?	Oberdisse et al. 1980
	Saarland 1974	2.40	?	Oberdisse et al. 1980
	Saarland 1983	1.90	1.40	Kurihara et al. 1984
	Average 1983	1.60	1.78	
Germany, GDR	Average	1.4	2.0	Kurihara et al. 1984
Hongkong	Average	3.05	2.6	Kurihara et al. 1984
Hungary	Szaboles	1.25	2.8	Kurihara et al. 1984
	Vas	0.85	1.85	
	Average	1.05	2.3	
Iceland	Average	4.35	3.82	Stanbury, Hetzel 1980
India	Bombay	1.4	1.8	Kurihara et al. 1984
	Poona	1.2	4.5	
	Average	1.3	3.15	
Israel	Average 1982	4.2	2.6	Kurihara et al. 1984
	Average 1974	1.9	2.2	Oberdisse et al. 1980 Stanbury, Hetzel 1980

Table 6 (continued)

Country	Area	Incidence/ 100000/year	Females/ males	Source
Italy	Varese	3.7	2.2	Kurihara et al. 1984
Jamaica	Kingston	2.1	2.4	Kurihara et al. 1984
Japan	Fukuoka	1.55	2.1	Kurihara et al. 1984
	Miyagi	1.85	2.7	Stanbury, Hetzel 1980
	Nagano	130 (?)	?	Hedinger 1969
	Nagasaki	4.75	3.3	Kurihara et al. 1984
	Osaka	1.15	2.8	Kurihara et al. 1984
Mozambique	Lourenco-Marques	2.05	1.4	Stanbury, Hetzel 1980
Netherlands	5 provinces	1.75	2.58	Stanbury, Hetzel 1980
New Zealand	Maori	4.7	3.92	Kurihara et al. 1984
	Non Maori	2.15	2.58	
Nigeria	Ibadan	2.15	4.35	Stanbury, Hetzel 1984
Norway	Average 1984	2.95	2.93	Kurihara et al. 1984
	Average 1973	3.24	?	Oberdisse et al. 1980
	Average 1969	1.50	2.0	Hedinger 1969
Poland	Szczecin	1.48	1.9	Kurihara et al. 1984
	Cracow	1.60	1.47	
	Katowice	0.85	1.42	
	Nowy Sacz	2.0	0.9	
	Warsaw	1.45	2.61	
	Average	1.48	1.66	
Romania	Cluj County	0.95	3.75	Kurihara et al. 1984
Senegal	Dakar	0.85	1.84	Kurihara et al. 1984
Singapore	Average 1984	2.49	2.42	Kurihara et al. 1984
	Chinese	0.75	2.0	Stanbury, Hetzel 1980
South Africa	Johannesbourg (Bantu)	0.9 (?)	17.0 (?)	Stanbury, Hetzel 1980
Spain	Navarra	1.2	2.42	Kurihara et al. 1984
	Zaragoza	3.3	4.50	
	Average	2.25	3.45	
Sweden	Average	2.65	2.46	Kurihara et al. 1984
Switzerland	Genève	2.80	1.67	Kurihara et al. 1984
	Neuchâtel	2.85	3.75	
	Vaud	2.95	3.90	
	Average	2.86	3.11	
Uganda	Kyadondo	1.35	26.0 (?)	Stanbury, Hetzel 1980
United Kingdom	Average 1963	3.0	?	Oberdisse et al. 1980
	England & Wales (4 regions)	0.85	2.4	Stanbury, Hetzel 1980
	Scotland average	1.21	2.16	Kurihara et al. 1984
	Average 1984	1.11	2.28	
USA	Bay Area	4.5	2.8	Kurihara et al. 1984
	Los Angeles	3.75	3.1	
	Connecticut	3.1	2.26	
	New York State	2.7	2.18	
	Puerto Rico	1.9	3.21	
	Hawaii 1984	10.3 (!)	2.81	
	Hawaii 1969	5.35	1.84	Hedinger 1969
Yugoslavia	Slovenia	1.9	1.24	Stanbury, Hetzel 1980

that thyroid cancer is mostly a very impressive disease in endemic goiter regions (Fig. 2), while it often shows up in a somewhat mitigated form in goiter free countries. As also mentioned, the prognosis of thyroid cancer is generally worse in regions with endemic goiter. This fact can be explained by 2 important factors:

a) In endemic goiter countries nobody is primarily worried by the growth of a "lump in the neck", such a feature is considered as "a normal development" until serious symptoms of the disease occur: Dyspnea due to tracheal compression or pulmonary metastases, dysphagia due to invasion of the esophagus, pain due to nerve irritation or bone metastases etc. It is therefore a frequent observation, that thyroid cancer patients in endemic goiter areas are first seen only in advanced tumor stages (Table 7), which – of course – impairs chances for a radical cure and increases mortality due to the disease.
b) In general highly aggressive histological tumor types are present in a large part of thyroid cancer cases from endemic goiter areas, while prognostically more favourable tumors prevail in goiter free countries (see Table 15). As we know (Waldhart 1963), that the histological tumor type is closely related to the prognosis of the disease, a high incidence of biologically "mean" thyroid cancer forms will also contribute to the relatively bad prognosis of thyroid malignancy in endemic goiter zones. In general, therefore, even as overall incidence of thyroid cancer does not seem to be related to iodine deficiency and/or endemic goiter, the outcome of the disease is certainly worse in such areas, due to a high incidence of "hopeless malignancies" (Huber, Riccabona 1967) either defined by histological tumor type or tumor stage.

Case K.A., 49.25.12.15, female, 54 years

Previous history: surgery for benign endemic goiter 1939. End of september 1969 rapid growth of recurrent goiter, hoarseness, pain on the right side of the neck, weakness, weight loss, admission to our hospital on october 22nd, 1969: inspiratory stridor, very firm, nodular and tender recurrent goiter on the right with reduced mobility (nodule diameter ~ 10 cm), pulse 80/min., BP 130/70, physical exam otherwise normal. Other findings: BSR 45/83, 81% Hb, 43 Vol% Htc, 12800 WBC. Recurrent nerve paralysis on the right side, no thyroid

Table 7. TNM stages of thyroid cancer in an endemic goiter area before and after iodized salt prophylaxis in comparison to a goiter free zone

Japan	$T_{0-2}N_0M_0$ 51.8%	$T_{0-2}N_{1,2}M_0$ 11.8%	$T_{3,4}N_3M_1$ 36.4%
Austria 1972	19.2%	9.8%	71.0%
Austria 1978	34.8%	4.8%	60.4%
Austria 1983 [a]	67.5%	5.6%	26.9%

[a] 20 years after introduction of iodized salt

autoantibodies. Moderate tracheal compression from 17 to 14 mm, but widening of retrotracheal space on X-ray films. ^{131}I-thyroid scan: Cold nodule on the right side. Course: right thyroid lobectomy on october 31st, 1969 (presumably radical). Histology: malignant hemangioendothelioma. On the 5th day postop. bloody secretion from the otherwise normally healing wound, increasing over the following days. On the 8th postop. day therefore revision of the neck with removal of large blood clots, hemostasis and macroscopic suspicion of tumor recurrence. Histology negative. After another 5 days again bleeding from the wound, blood units were given, coagulation parameters normal. Increasing swelling of neck and dyspnea. Therefore 2nd surgical revision of the neck on november 20th, 1969: blood clots removed again, hemostasis, obviously recurrent tumor with infiltration of trachea and larynx. Histology: positive. Once more after another 5 days bleeding from the wound, exulcerating tumor recurrence in the following days, no evidence of metastasis. Because of acute asphyxia tracheostomy in preterminal condition through huge necrotic tumor masses on december 23rd, 1969. Death from cardiac arrest on december 24th, 1969. Summary: extremely aggressive thyroid cancer (hemangioendothelioma) which killed the patient despite intense therapy in 3 months since the first symptoms.

3 Genetic Influences on Epidemiology of Thyroid Cancer

Even though overall genetic factors in the epidemiology of cancer contribute only relatively few cases (~ 1,6%) in our material, the fact that such influences do exist and can well be recognized is an interesting feature of thyroid malignancy and also presents more questions than answers.

Medullary Thyroid Carcinoma (MTC) in the Context of the Multiple Endocrine Neoplasia Syndrome (MEN)

Since years it has been known that such thyroid tumors occur in families, which also show other neoplastic transformations in different endocrine organs (Williams 1979). A correlation of medullary thyroid carcinoma with phaeochromocytoma (Baylin et al. 1976) serotonine-secreting intestinal neuromas and parathyroid adenomas as well as other typical clinical findings is observed occasionally in one family and screening by laboratory tests and/or CT, ultrasound etc. has revealed a remarkably high incidence of "latent" MEN-cases in such genetic lines. As aetiology of thyroid cancer will be discussed in a later chapter it should just be mentioned in the epidemiological section that medullary thyroid cancer cases should trigger a careful screening of the patient's family restricted not only to the diagnosis of thyroid lesions but also to the detection of other disorders in the framework of MEN. This can help to start appropriate therapy in due time and may provide a guideline to genetic counseling, as it is well known that this syndrome is transmitted genetically in a dominant way (Williams 1981).

Other Genetic Influences

Concerning tumor types other than medullary carcinoma the evidence of genetic influences on the epidemiology of the disease is scattered in the literature (Weinstein, Kitchin 1971) and often remains restricted to case reports (Riccabona et al. 1983). It is remarkable, however, that both twins in which an endogenous genetically determined defect of thyroid hormone synthesis was reported first (Stanbury, Hedge 1950) were later victims of thyroid cancer. Thus, the question arises again if genetic goitrogenic influences can also stimulate the growth of thyroid cancer. Taking endemic goiter as an example, it was demonstrated that in the same iodine deficient environment genetic influences do play a significant role in goitrogenesis (Table 8) (Bauer et al. 1973). The molecular basis of such factors was studied partly (Riccabona 1972, Platzer et al. 1980) but conclusive evidence of the primary disorder in thyroid cell growth and metabolism is still lacking (Stanbury, Hetzel 1980). Perhaps the recent reports on thyroid-growth-stimulating-immunoglobulins, on the interaction of TSH with receptors and cAMP-metabolism in certain cell clones can provide further information in the future. It should be stressed in this context, that among our own patients 1,5% belonged to "thyroid cancer families" (Riccabona et al. 1983). An impressive example of a pedigree is shown in Fig. 3. These observations far exceed the statistical probability of coincidences of thyroid cancer in 2 generations ($p = < 0.05$). Obviously therefore genetical influences can play a role in the epidemiology of thyroid cancer in general, the specific nature of these factors is, however, not adequately understood at present.

Epidemiology of Thyroid Cancer Related to Autoimmune Thyroid Disease

For decades a correlation between chronic thyroiditis (Hashimoto's disease) and thyroid cancer has been discussed (Lindsay 1960). More specifically malignant thyroid lymphoma seemed to occur with increased frequency in patients with Hashimoto's disease (Dinsmore et al. 1949). Another important observation was made in thyroid glands removed because of Graves' disease: It was found that sclerosing papillary microcarcinomas of the Graham type (Shapiro et al. 1970) were found sometimes in these specimens even as only very few pa-

Table 8. Genetic influence for goitrogenesis in endemic goiter

Maladaption to iodine deficiency	Partial enzyme insufficiency Partial trapping defect Inadequate thyroglobulin	
Autoimmunity disorders	Thyroid growth stimulating Autoantibodies	
I-deficiency (urinary I/g creat. ca. 35 μg)	Goiter incidence Parents goitrous No parent goitrous	 44.9% 16.6%

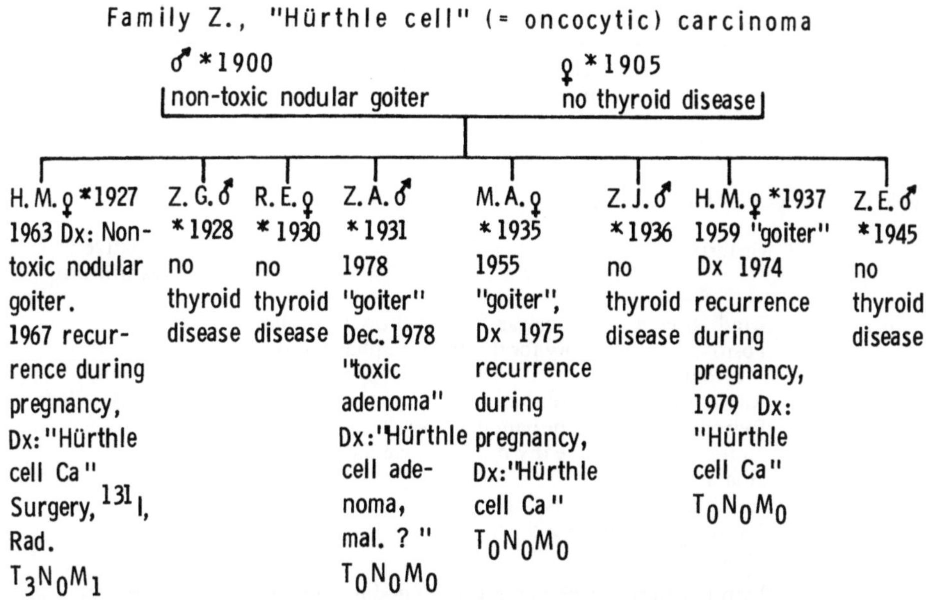

Fig. 3. Pedigree of family with 4 Huerthle-cell tumors in one generation. Another Family (ZE) with 3 follicular carcinomas in one generation is now also known in our series

tients showed the clinical course of thyroid malignancy (Hazard et al. 1949). It was also reported that intense lymphocytic infiltration around a thyroid carcinoma would improve the prognosis of the disease (Goudie 1968). Finally we are confronted today with the existence of "thyroid growth stimulating immunoglobulins" (Chiovato et al. 1984), which might also be implicated in the pathogenesis of thyroid cancer. At present, however, there is no adequate evidence to relate thyroid autoimmune disorders such as chronic thyroiditis of the Hashimoto type or Graves' disease with the epidemiology of thyroid cancer with the exception of malignant thyroid lymphoma. In these cases the sequence of the underlying pathology is still a matter of discussion (Heimann et al. 1978). Without taking into account the possible significance of thyroid growth stimulating autoantibodies, the overall impact of thyroid autoimmune disorders on the epidemiology of thyroid cancers seems to be rather small.

Summary

In addition to the epidemiological factors mentioned above it should be noted, that we observed a significantly high incidence of thyroid carcinoma in couples (Table 9) (Riccabona et al. 1983). Radiation exposure and other familial oncogenic factors were ruled out in our studies. Viral and/or unknown environmental factors in the pathogenesis of these thyroid cancers cannot, however, be ruled out. Overall therefore thyroid cancer shows no obvious correlation to endemic goiter in it's incidence although iodine deficiency seems to

Table 9. Thyroid cancer in couples (own material – observation period 6 yrs.)

Thyroid cancer	Thyroid cancer in couples	Significance
n=450	n=8	p=<0.01

Table 10. Risk groups for thyroid cancer

	Criteria	Relative significance [a]
History	Irradiation of head, neck and upper chest in childhood	++
	Positive family history for thyroid Ca., phaeochromocytoma etc.	++
	Rapid growth of thyroid nodule	+++
	Retroauricular pain or pain in goiter	+
	Goiter growth inspite thyroid hormone therapy	+++
	Hoarseness	+
	Rapid growth <20 yrs.	+++
	Rapid goiter growth > 50 yrs.	+++
	Dyspnea	+
Physical exam	Lymph nodes in neck in presence of nodular goiter	++
	Firm thyroid nodule with irregular outline	+++
	Thyroid nodule with infiltration of surrounding structures	+++
	Spontaneous recurrent nerve paralysis in presence of nodular goiter	++
Other results	Cold nodule in thyroid scan	+
	Hypodense echo structure in thyroid nodule with irregular outline	+
	Fine needle biopsy Pap. III – Pap. V	+++
	^{131}I-uptake in metastases	+++
	Serum-thyroglobulin > 30 ng/ml	+
	Calcitonin 500 pg/ml	+++
	Elevated BSR	+
	Radiological evidence of metastases in presence of nodular goiter	+
		43+=total

[a] Highly suspicious above 14+

impair the prognosis of the disease. Genetic influences in the epidemiology of thyroid malignancy exist as well as environmental influences of an unknown nature (except ionizing radiation as a known pathogenetic factor). Females are afflicted more frequently by these tumors than males and in general thyroid cancer has it's peak incidence after the 4th decade. In trying to establish risk groups according to the epidemiological data mentioned previously a pattern can be established for general purposes as shown in Table 10.

Thyroid Cancer and other Diseases

With the exception of the familial form of medullary carcinoma in the MEN-syndrome and a correlation between generalized malignant lymphomas and thyroid manifestations of this disorder very little is known regarding coincidences of extrathyroidal disease with thyroid cancer (Alderson 1980, Ellenberg et al. 1962). Old reports exist on tuberculosis of the thyroid but no evidence of malignancy was found in these cases. There are, however, some notes suggesting a relationship between thyroid disease and breast cancer (Schottenfeld, Berg 1971) and there are even some cases with breast cancer and thyroid cancer seen by us and others (Schottenfeld, Gersham 1977). So far the statistical validity of these observations remains not quite convincing. Occupational possibly carcinogenic factors do not provide an increased risk of thyroid malignancy with the exception of work with ionizing radiation.

Obviously there are "high risk groups" within "risk groups in general" and all these details should be considered in selecting the diagnostic approach to an individual patient.

Pathology of Thyroid Cancer

1 Conventional Classifications

As mentioned previously many authors have described histological types of thyroid cancer since decades. The classification of thyroid neoplasms finally became so confusing that the International Union against Cancer (UICC) together with the World Health Organization (WHO) decided to tackle this problem and therefore a "new classification" of thyroid cancer was established (Hedinger, Sobin 1974). It has been widely accepted (Table 11) all over the world, because it helps pathologists in their difficult task of making a definite diagnosis, even as many centers feel, that the actual classification is missing several details (Hedinger 1983). The evolution of the actual classification is shown in Table 12 and in the context of this publication it does not seem justified to present the well-known classical examples of different tumor types, which can be studied in any textbook of pathology (Waldhart 1969). The discussion whether the actually valid classification of thyroid cancer types should also be accepted in the future, goes on in the scientific community (Williams 1980). Do a few papillae in a mixed thyroid tumor indeed justify the diagnosis of papillary carcinoma? Are onkocytic thyroid neoplasms essentially malignant? Where is the border between malignancy and benign thyroid adenomas, when no invasion of the vessels and/or capsule can be shown? (Fig. 4). Is medullary thyroid carcinoma

Table 11. WHO-classification of thyroid tumors

I)		Epithelial tumors	II)	Non-epithelial
A)		Benign:	A)	Benign
	1)	Follicular Adenoma	B)	Malignant
	2)	Other		Fibrosarcoma
				Others
B)		Malignant		
	1)	Follicular Ca	III)	Various tumors
	2)	Papillary Ca	1)	Carcinosarcoma
	3)	Squamous cell Ca	2)	Malignant hemangioendothelioma
	4)	Anaplastic Ca		
	a)	Spindle cell type	3)	Malignant lymphoma
	b)	Giant cell type	4)	Teratoma
	c)	Small cell type	IV)	Metastases
	5)	Medullary Ca	V)	Unclassified tumors
			VI)	Tumor-like changes

Table 12. Older classifications of thyroid cancer

Langhans, Wegelin, quoted by Walthard		Crile, Hazard, Dinsmore	
1)	*Epithelial Forms*	A	Carcinoma
a)	"Metastasizing adenoma"	I)	Papillary
b)	Onkozytic metastasizing adenoma	II)	Not papillary
c)	Proliferating goiter "Langhans"	a)	Angioinvasive Adenoma
d)	Papilloma	b)	Adeno-Ca.
e)	Solid carcinoma, squamous cell, cylindrocellular	c)	Undiff. Ca.
		III)	Special Types
2)	*Sarcomas*	a)	Non encapsulated sclerosing Tu. (Graham)
a)	Without intercellular material (spindle cell, polymorph cell, giant cell, round cell sarcoma)	b)	Squamous cell Ca.
		c)	Metastatic Ca.
b)	With collagene intercellular material (fibro-myxo-osteochondro-sarcoma)	B	Sarcoma
3)	Hemangioendothelioma	I)	Lymphosarcomas
4)	Carcino-sarcoma	II)	Spindle cell sarcoma

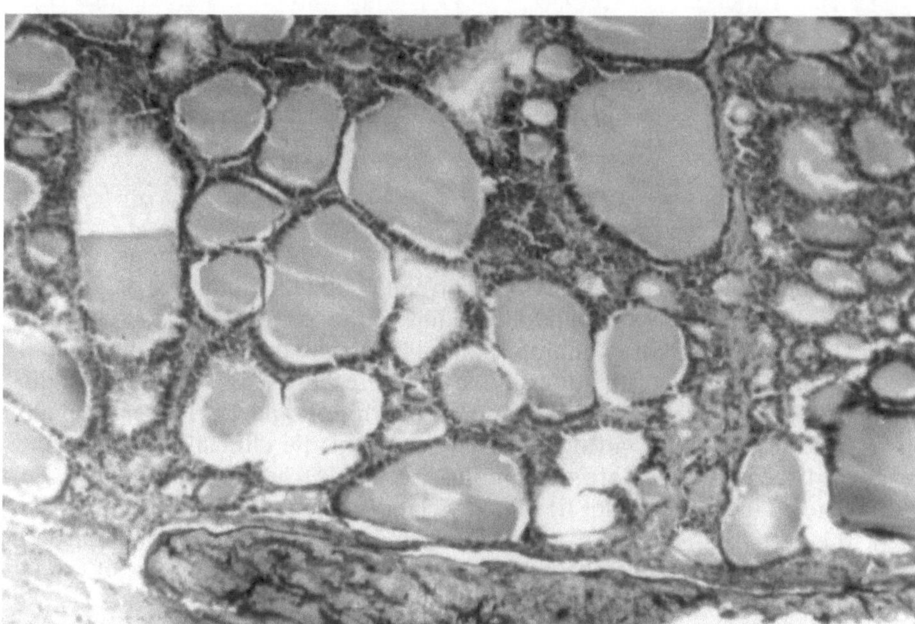

Fig. 4. "Metastazing Adenoma" = Skull metastasis of well differentiated follicular thyroid carcinoma. Without adjacent bone structures the histological pattern could be classified as macrofollicular nodular goiter and no diagnosis of malignancy would be apparent

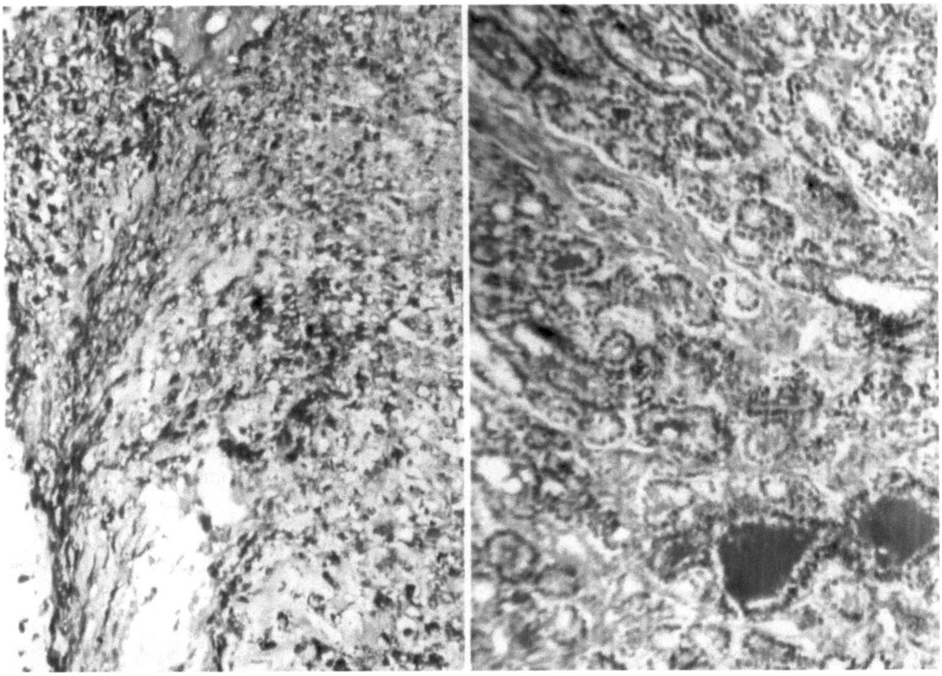

Fig. 5. Histology sections of patient with large thyroid cancer. Structures of badly differentiated follicular thyroid carcinoma, anaplastic carcinoma (spindle cell) and sarcoma (cartilage!) within the same lesion!

really and always only a tumor of the C-cell system? Are squamous cell carcinomas "metaplastic" alterations of a primary adeno-carcinoma of the thyroid? Are malignant hemangioendotheliomas of the thyroid really sarcomas or should they be classified as angioplastic, anaplastic carcinomas (Thaler et al. 1986)? Are lymphomas of the thyroid local manifestations of a generalized disease or do they represent a special tumor in the thyroid gland? These and many other questions are still waiting for answers. From the clinical point of view, however, it seems that we are demanding too much from the pathologist: Tumors as shown in Fig. 5 do not fit into any classification and the clinician has to accept the fact, that the most aggressive tumor sections in such mixed neoplasms in general are the "pacemakers" for the biological behaviour of the lesion (Ibanez et al. 1966).

Nevertheless the actually valid histopathological classification of thyroid cancer can be regarded as an important progress for clinicians and pathologists all over the world, as it has established internationally accepted criteria for the diagnosis of thyroid malignancy and as it therefore makes epidemiological studies possible that could never have been realized with the older classifications.

There is another problem regarding histopathology which has also been mentioned above: The histological tumor pattern can change with time so that

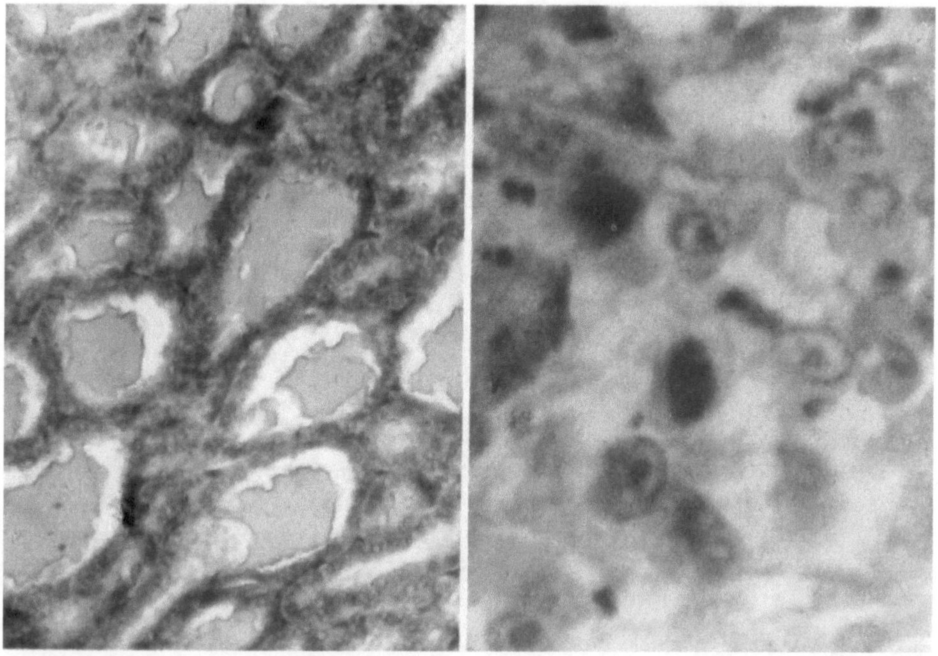

Fig. 6. Histology of patient with follicular thyroid Ca. (lung metastasis) responding well to ^{131}I-therapy over many years (*left*). Another metastasis developed after 5 years in the pelvis without ^{131}I-uptake, rapid progression which finally was responsible for death. Histology shows an anaplastic tumor (*right*)

frequently primarily well-differentiated adeno-carcinomas become anaplastic tumors (Fig. 6). It is also known (Riccabona 1972) that metastases can show a quite different histology than the primary lesion. Thus, any histopathological classification should be considered as relevant only for a certain tumor localization and for a given time.

Certain improvements regarding histopathological diagnosis in thyroid tumors have also been obtained with semithin sections, while we have the impression that normal frozen sections can provide adequate diagnosis if they are done by experienced pathologists (Schauer 1984) (Fig. 7).

The possibility to measure DNA in thyroid tissue by Feulgen-cytophotometry is an important tool for studying thyroid cell metabolism in tissue specimens (Table 13). These data can be obtained today partly with the help of automated counting systems and give us significant information concerning the proliferative activity of thyroid cells (Hofstädter et al. 1983). While highly aggressive thyroid cancer shows therefore definitely increased DNA-values, the difference between benign adenomas and well differentiated thyroid carcinoma remains mostly unsignificant, so that such DNA-measurements in thyroid tumors can only give "adjunctive knowledge" on growth tendencies in such lesions and will frequently not be adequate to draw the borderline between benign and malignant thyroid nodules.

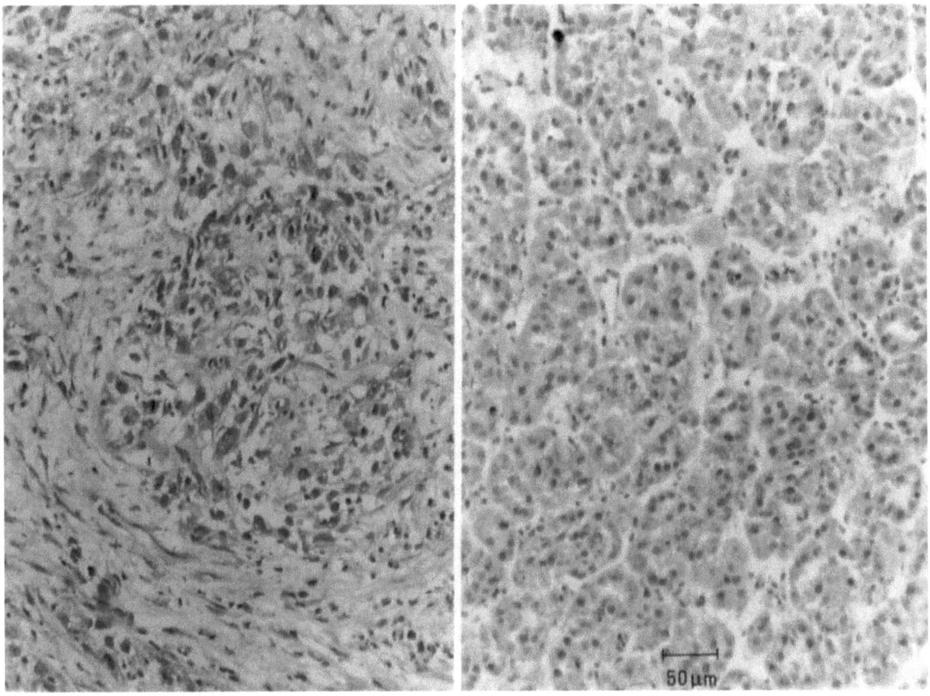

Fig. 7. Frozen sections of aggressive thyroid cancer (*left*) and well differentiated thyroid carcinoma (*right*), which can be recognized only by demonstration of invasive growth

Table 13. DNA-Feulgen cytophotometry in benign and malignant thyroid nodules: DNA-tumor-stemlines of 25 removed cold nodules

	2c	2c<x<4c	4c	n
Adenomas	8 (73%)	2 (18%)	1 (9%)	11 (100%)
Carcinomas	4 (29%)	6 (42%)	4 (29%)	14 (100%)
n	12 (48%)	8 (32%)	5 (20%)	25 (100%)

A variety of other cytochemical methods can of course help in the classification of thyroid malignancy. Congo red reacts with small proteins in the amyloid stroma containing also calcitonin in medullary thyroid carcinoma (Waldhart 1969). Techniques to establish the real nature of fibrous material can improve the distinction between sarcomatous lesions and other fibrous changes in thyroid nodules, which can partly be due to scar formation or to chronic thyroiditis. Sudan stains reveal lipids in thyroid nodules, which can either occur as manifestations of degeneration in partly necrotic tissue or as an element of the very rare thyrolipoma (Fig. 8) (Schroeder et al. 1984).

Without making any claim that this short chapter on the pathology of thyroid cancer is a detailed review of the relevant and very complex problem at hand, it should rather present difficulties and the potential possibilities for

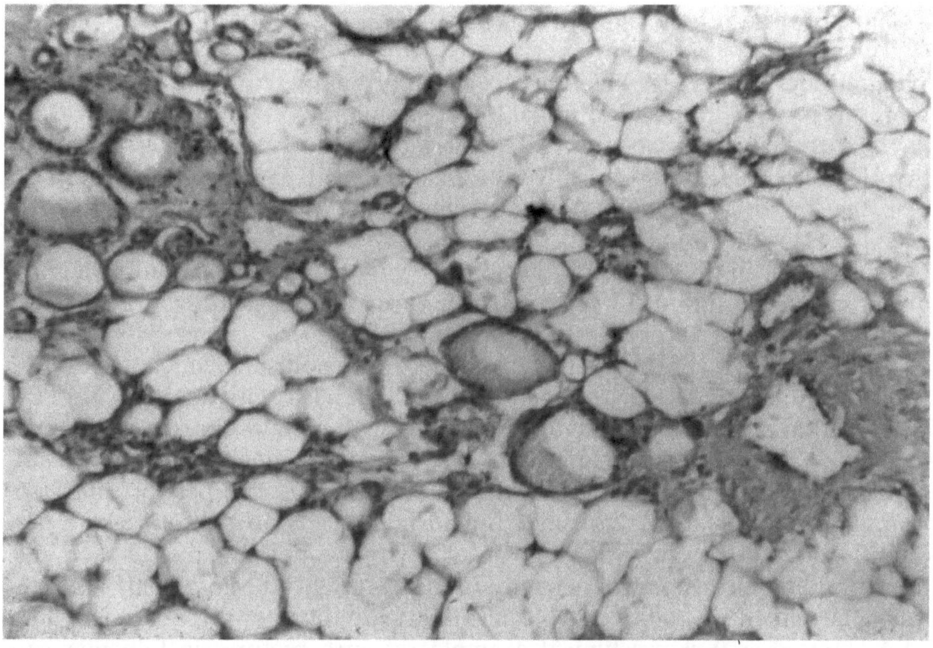

Fig. 8. Histology of "Thyrolipoma", presenting clinically as malignant thyroid nodule

pathologists, when clinicians want to understand the pecularities of one thyroid cancer in one given patient.

It should be stressed, however, that recent advances in histopathological techniques as described later on may – in the future – modify the current concepts of pathology of thyroid cancer and provide us with better criteria concerning the nature of different thyroid tumors.

Finally it should be mentioned that a variety of malignant tumors can (Walther 1948) develop metastases in the thyroid gland. These, of course, suggest clinically malignant goiters. Hypernephroid renal carcinomas can develop thyroidal metastases which are sometimes interpreted wrongly as "clear cell carcinoma" of the thyroid. In patients with known malignancies of other organs, any rapidly developing thyroid nodule should primarily be considered as a metastasis of the original neoplasm (Shimaoka et al. 1962) and diagnostic as well as therapeutic approaches should take this possibility into account.

A few cases are known also, in which a "struma ovarii" showed malignant development (Mayberger 1959). These ovarian abnormalities must be classified as specifically organized teratomas and not as thyroid cancer per se. Malignant development can also occur in dystopic thyroids (Fish, Moore 1963).

2 Immunohistochemical Findings

The immuno peroxydase reaction in slices (normal or semithin) of thyroid tumors has provided much additional information on the pathophysiological behaviour of such lesions and has added a new dimension to our understanding of thyroid cancer and to it's classification (Caillou et al. 1983). The development of potent antibodies against thyroglobulin, calcitonin, CEA, somatostatin and even ACTH resulted in microscopic pictures showing well defined antigen-antibody reactions in the tissues of different thyroid neoplasms and thus even produced insights in the different roles of a variety of subcellular structures for pathophysiological abnormalities within thyroid cancer (Thomas-Morvan et al. 1974). It will be mentioned later, that these immunohistochemical techniques can be combined with electron microscopy which has improved even more the coordination of immunoperoxydase reactions with certain ultrastructural components of thyroid tissue (Hofstädter 1983). Today with the increasing availability of monoclonal antibodies to many antigens it seems possible that conventional concepts of thyroid cancer might be replaced in the future by a new classification which allows a "typing" of thyroid neoplasms due to their different immunohistochemical behaviour (Klinck 1969). The commonly used immunohistochemical studies involve anti-thyroglobulin, anti-calcitonin and anti-CEA stains. Fig. 9 shows typical examples of such pictures in follicular carcinoma and medullary carcinoma. On the basis of such studies it was possible to show that medullary carcinoma is obviously not such a well-defined tumor as postulated in the past, but that such lesions can produce thyroglobulin as well as calcitonin and CEA (Pfaltz et al. 1983). It was also reported, that "anaplastic" thyroid carcinomas can show thyroglobulin formation as a proof of some degree of functional differentiation. With specific immunohistochemical reactions (precreatin, vimentine) the classification of malignant thyroid lymphomas and so-called "small-cell" carcinoma of the thyroid has also changed significantly (Schauer 1984). Positive immunohistochemical stains with factor 8 in "hemangioendothelioma" seem to support the old hypothesis that this is indeed a sarcoma and a special pathological entity and not just a modification of anaplastic carcinoma (Hedinger 1983, Thaler et al. 1986). Rare malignant lesions in the thyroid such as paraganglioma, malignant fibrous histocytomas can frequently also be recognized with the help of modern immunohistochemical methods. At present a tentative pattern of immunohistochemical tumor types in the thyroid might be proposed as shown in Table 14. Whether such a

Table 14. Immunohistochemical criteria for classification of thyroid carcinoma

	Hemangioendothelioma	Diff. thyroid Ca.	Anaplastic thyroid Ca.	Medull. thyroid Ca.	Lymphoma
Thyroglobulin	−	+	±	+	−
Calcitonin	−	−	−	+	−
Somatostatin	−	−	−	+	−
Lymphocyte antigen	−	−	−	−	+
Factor VIII	+	−	−	−	−

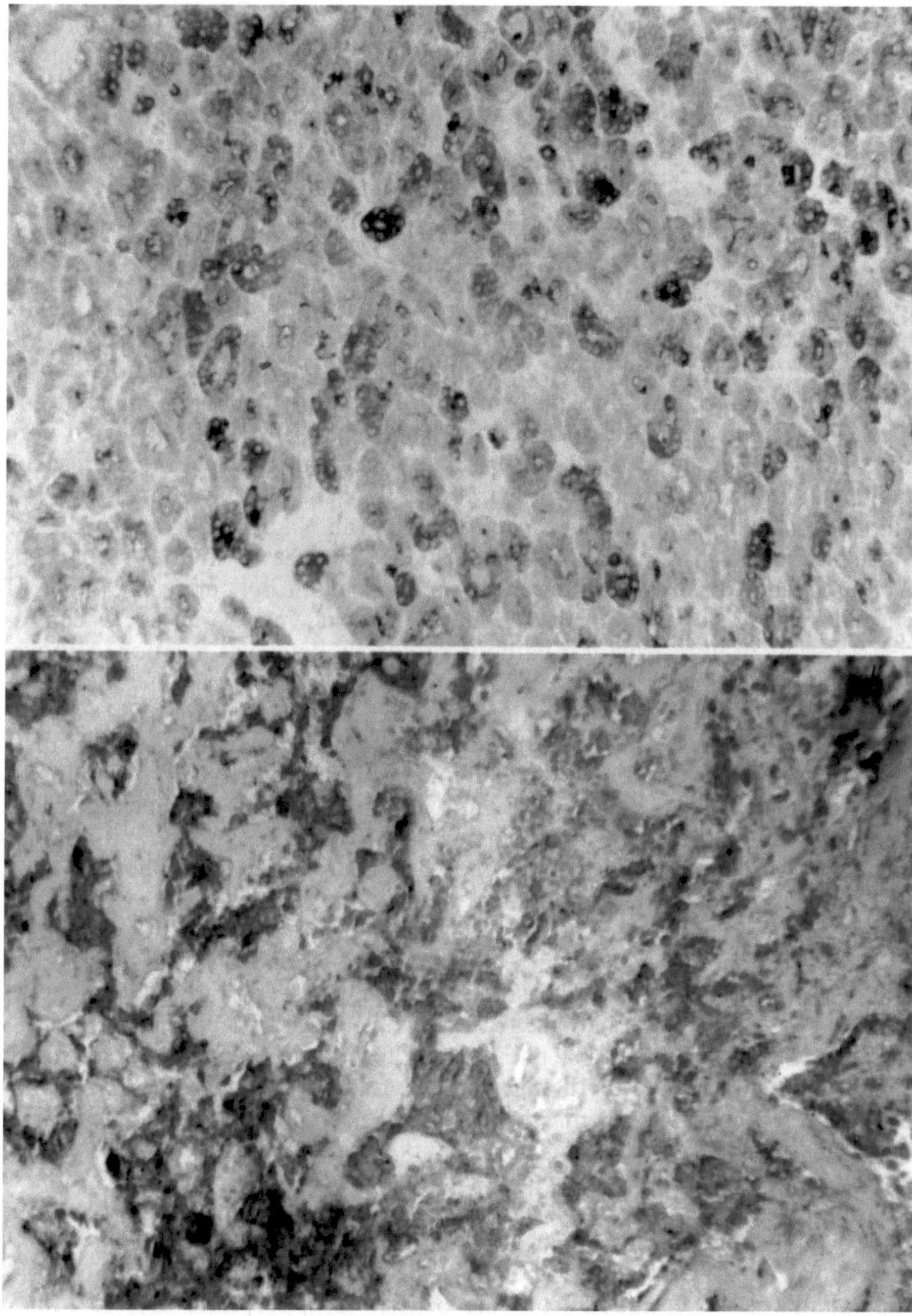

Fig. 9. Immunohistochemistry: differentiated thyroid cancer with thyroglobulin staining (*above*) and medullary thyroid carcinoma with positive calcitonine-reaction (*below*)

classification is really an important progress in our understanding of thyroid malignancy and therefore in our therapeutic approach will be known only in the future and certainly only together with all the other informations gathered with new pathological techniques.

3 Electron Microscopy

Even though ordinary light microscopy provides us with quick and frequently reliable diagnoses of thyroid tumors, immunohistochemistry and electron microscopy are recognized by now as techniques which – with additional costs, skilled performance and some patience – provide more details for clinicians on the structure and nature of such lesions (Jao, Gold 1975). Usually fixed with glutaraldehyde and embedded in Durcupan specimens for electron microscopy can be studied either as native preparations, they can also be studied with immunohistochemistry, Feulgen cytophotometry and autoradiography. Native pictures permit a differentiation of subcellular structures in thyroid tumor cells such as colloid droplets, mitochondria, endoplasmatic reticulum and signs of pinocytosis (Fig. 10) (Ekholm 1964). Immunohistochemical approaches can reveal a variety of ultrastructural pathophysiological details as mentioned above. The same is true concerning DNA-Feulgen cytophotometry. Microautoradiography – be it of live tumors or tumor cell cultures – can also provide important information on the biological behaviour of thyroid neoplasia. Using either ^{125}I or compounds associated with malignant cell development (e.g. ^{3}H-Thymidine, labeled TSH etc.) (Winand, Kohn 1975) pictures can be obtained which are frequently impressive in their diagnostic impact (Fig. 11). The information gathered with such techniques underlines the facts reported previously:

"Anaplastic" thyroid carcinomas can show "colloid droplets" as manifestations of functional properties, subcellular elements considered as typical of medullary carcinoma can be detected in "adeno-carcinomas" of the thyroid (Pfaltz et al. 1983) and some ultrastructural elements seen in thyroid cancer resemble those observed in benign thyroid disease (Dinstl, Keminger 1967). At present therefore these refined pathological techniques seem to deliver many interesting scientific data on the nature of thyroid malignancy and can in some cases offer explanations for discrepancies between classical pathological definition and biological behaviour of a thyroid cancer. As stated in an earlier chapter it might well be, however, that in the future these studies could establish criteria for a new classification of thyroid cancer which would be useful for the choice between different therapeutic strategies. If such criteria should be acknowledged world-wide it must be accepted, that a majority of the world population will be excluded from the benefit of appropriate thyroid tumor classifications due to the small number of pathology departments capable of performing all the costly and sophisticated studies in developing countries. This will leave the clinician in such areas with the question, which therapeutic program should be considered in an individual case with regard to histopathology.

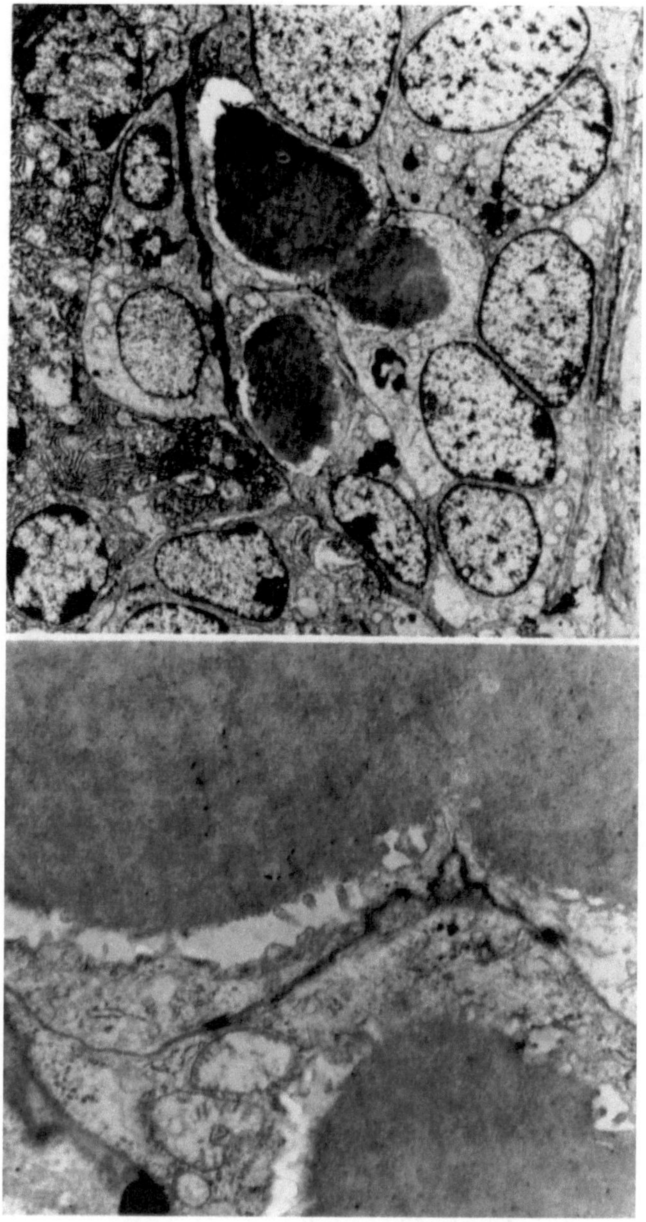

Fig. 10. Electron microscopy of thyroid cancer: *above:* intracellular colloid droplets in otherwise anaplastic thyroid carcinoma. *below:* condensed alveolar macrophage in anaplastic Ca

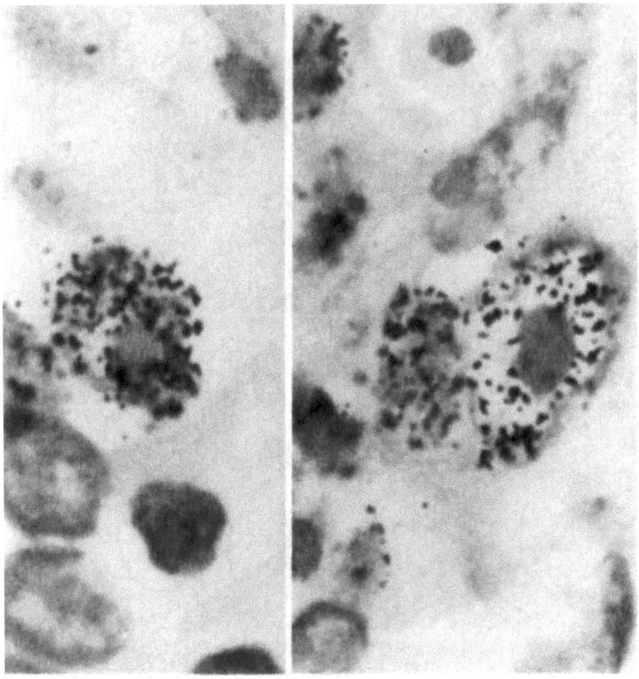

Fig. 11. Autoradiogram of cells of anaplastic thyroid Ca after incubation with ^{3}H-thymidine. Intense labeling of nuclei sparing nucleoli (exposure 10 days)

4 Correlation of Pathological Findings with Clinical Prognosis

Since thyroid cancer became known more widely pathologists and clinicians alike have been struck by the different biological behaviour of various thyroid neoplasms (Franssila 1971). Some authors (Clute, Warren 1935) suggested to define certain lesions as "hopeless malignancies", others as "definitely malignant but not hopeless" and a further group als "potentially malignant". The problems of all such approaches are perhaps outlined best in a case history (Huber, Riccabona 1967).

Case A.G., female, 52 years, 1967

1950 excision of bilateral lymph nodes in the neck. Histology: metastases of papillary thyroid carcinoma. 1951 radical surgery of thyroid and neck nodes. 1955 during pregnancy (interrupted) lung metastases demonstrated by chest film. Since then another pregnancy (uneventful), child healthy, patient doing well, lung foci without progression. Neck free.

Of course immunological and hormonal factors could be quoted to explain the clinical course of this patient. We also know that well-differentiated papillary carcinomas generally behave quite differently in young patients and in patients above 40 years of age:

Case K.M., 44.16.04.10, male, 58 years

Thyroid surgery 1923, postoperatively unilateral recurrent nerve paralysis. Because of increasing dyspnoea and hoarseness since October 1968 admission to ENT service on November 20th, 1968. Diagnosis: bilateral vocal chord paralysis. On exam moderate firm recurrent goiter (I) on the right side, which was "warm" on a 131 I-scan. BSR 21/36, radiography of chest and neck: narrowing of the trachea from 28 to 15 mm from the right with displacement of the trachea to the left, chest regular. As the patient had a myocardial infarction 3 years before it was decided to treat him with 32 mCi of ^{131}I on December 2nd, 1968 to avoid surgery if possible, but a tracheostomy was performed. In March 1969 radicular pain in the chest, x-rays reveal multiple metastases in thoracic spine and an osteolysis in the 8th rib on the right side. Widening of retrotracheal space. After symptomatic radiotherapy on the spine, right hemithyroidectomy on May 21st, 1969. Histology: papillary carcinoma. Thereafter 100 mCi ^{131}I on June 2nd, 1969. Then pleural effusion due to pleural carcinosis, rapid deterioration, death on June 24th, 1969 with disseminated metastases. Summary: highly aggressive papillary thyroid carcinoma in patient of 58 years with recurrent goiter with a span of 8 months from onset of symptoms to death in spite of therapy.

Case E.V., 20.06.03.51, female, 23 years

Autumn 1974 resection of an accidently detected lymphoma on right neck side. Histology: metastasis of papillary thyroid Ca. (mixed with follicular structures). December 3rd, 1974: Radical thyroidectomy with radical neck dissection on the right as other lymph nodes were palpable also. Histology positive. 60 Gy to neck in 2 series, 100 mCi of ^{131}I on June 23rd, 1975. Since then doing well, tumor free. Summary: primarily massive lymph node metastases to neck nodes from papillary carcinoma of the right lobe in young female, intense surgical and radiological therapy, probably cure after more than 10 years follow-up.

Small papillary tumors can present primarily by extensive lymph node involvement. When adequate therapy can be done, even such patients can definitely be cured. For decades, therefore, efforts were made to correlate pathological criteria of thyroid tumors with prognosis (Russel et al. 1975). Carefully done statistical analyses (Ladurner et al. 1984) do show some significant trends as outlined in Table 15. These "trends", however, should not be regarded as definite prognostic factors in each case. The usually very aggressive "squamous cell carcinoma" can also show a course as described in the next case history.

Case W.D., 98.05.10.12, female, 65 years

Rapid goiter growth, increasing dyspnoea since December 1976. February 26th 1977 therefore subtotal bilateral unradical thyroidectomy. Histology: squamous cell carcinoma of the left lobe. March 23rd, 1977: admission because of local

Table 15. Incidence and survival rates of different thyroid cancer types in goiter-free countries (according to Hedinger 1969) and an endemic goiter area (according to Riccabona, 1974)[a]

	Differentiated adeno-Ca.		Undifferentiated Ca.[b]		Other thyroid cancers[c]	
	Incidence (%)	5-yr survival (%)	Incidence (%)	5-yr survival (%)	Incidence (%)	5-yr survival (%)
Hedinger (1,456 cases)	72.8	75	1.9	16	25.3	3.13
Riccabona	56.2	69	28.4[d]	14	15.4[e]	0

[a] Problems of histological classification (see below) make comparison difficult, but comprehensive interpretation of the existing data was attempted.
[b] Anaplastic, small-, spindle, and giant-cell carcinomas, possibly classified by other pathologists as "sarcomas."
[c] Solid, medullary, epidermoid, and lymphomas, possibly classified by other pathologists as "sarcomas" and "undifferentiated carcinomas."
[d] Solid anaplastic carcinomas (possibly including medullary, epidermoid carcinomas).
[e] Sarcomas (probably including some small-, spindle-, and giant-cell carcinomas as well as lymphomas).

recurrence with severe tracheal compression (15 to 7 mm) and invasion of the oesophagus. After 4 sessions with 0.15 Gy each, acute asphyxia, partial removal of the recurrent tumor. Histology: anaplastic thyroid cancer. Continuation of percutaneous radiotherapy, chemotherapy with vincristine and adriamycine, 120 mCi ^{131}I on April 22nd, 1977. Radiation therapy stopped with total dose of 28 Gy because of oesophago-tracheal fistula. Chemotherapy continued. May 23rd, 1986: no complaints, obviously tumor free, no dyspnoea, no dysphagia, no tracheal impairment.

With all these skeptical remarks on correlation between pathology and clinical prognosis it must be stressed, however, that for practical purposes the basic histological tumor type should become a guideline for adequate therapy (Hedinger 1983). Nevertheless we do not accept the concept that e.g. a frozen-section diagnosis of "anaplastic carcinoma" or of sarcoma should lure the clinician into therapeutic nihilism such as restricting the surgical procedure to a simple "open biopsy". It should be accepted, that aggressive tumors also require aggressive therapy, that the intensity and choice of therapy, however, should be modified according to pathological findings. On the other hand it does not seem justified to treat "low grade" thyroid malignancies just like ordinary benign goiters. Therefore, when we are confronted with a thyroid cancer patient, pathological reports can provide approximate data on the probability of a long-term cure, they can also help to establish appropriate therapy plans but they cannot give an answer concerning the individual patient's fate also in view of – among other things – the therapeutical decisions derived from pathological criteria. Will the patient "respond" to specifically chosen treatments or will he not?

With all the new techniques in research and diagnosis of thyroid cancer we might hope, that even more specific treatment patterns can be developed. We should, however, be reluctant to place too much of the burden of responsibility for the management of thyroid cancer patients on pathologists, who – with all their skills, knowledge and techniques – examine a piece of thyroid tumor tissue at a given moment. The dialogue, begun long ago, between pathologists and clinicians regarding all the problems cited in this chapter should therefore continue as one party always raises questions, which the other cannot answer. It is certain, that without the modifications in therapeutic strategies provided by pathological parameters the survival rate of thyroid cancer patients would be much lower, than it is at present. When we will know more about what happens in a thyroid tumor and not just how it looks like (partly due to methods described above) we might also be able to correlate pathology even better with clinical findings.

Pathophysiology of Thyroid Cancer

It was already mentioned in the previous chapter that many pathophysiological features of thyroid cancer can be detected with the refined techniques of modern pathology. This still somehow morphological approach to pathophysiology should be complemented by frequently kinetic studies of tumor cell metabolism if we really want to understand what is happening in a thyroid cancer and why. It is generally accepted that 3 major advances in methodology have produced the most important informations on this topic in recent years:

a) The widespread use of radiotracers to study a variety of metabolic phenomena in tumor tissue and their dynamic behaviour (Pochin, Thompson 1969, Ackermann, Marvin 1961).
b) The developments of analytical chemistry in general and especially in protein chemistry which allow us to define also structural abnormalities in tumor tissue and
c) the possibility to use both methods for the study of thyroid cancer not only in patients or experimental animals, but also in cell cultures of certain types of thyroid neoplasms (Caviedes, Stanbury 1976).

The introduction of ^{131}I several decades ago provided the first important data on altered tissue function in thyroid cancer (Black et al. 1953). It was found that usually thyroid cancer had an impaired uptake of iodine and reduced iodide trapping capacity (Horst 1961), due to a functional dedifferentiation which is often correlated with the histological pattern (Horst, Heuwieser 1957). It was also noted (Edmonds et al. 1977) that iodine uptake could also be increased in thyroid carcinoma by TSH (Sturgeon et al. 1953), which implied several diagnostic and therapeutic possibilities for the management of the disease (Riccabona 1980). With ever improving diagnostic possibilities it was also reported that there were a few very well differentiated thyroid carcinomas with an increased radioiodine uptake when compared with normal surrounding thyroid tissue and with all the criteria of a "toxic nodule" (Abdel-Razzak, Christie 1979). The amount of thyroid hormone produced and stored even in metastases of thyroid carcinomas proved to be so high in a few cases, that high-dose ^{131}I-treatment of such lesions resulted in thyroid storm due to abrupt release of vast amounts of thyroid hormone from the damaged tumor tissue in the circulation (Raith et al. 1970). It was also found that the half-life of ^{131}I taken up in thyroid cancers was unusually short (Horst 1961) and relevant studies showed a discharge of non-organically bound iodine from tumor tissue as one factor for explanation of this phenomenon (Nieponemizce et al. 1969).

In general the amount of inactive iodine is also reduced in thyroid cancers according to data from fluorescent scanning (Patton et al. 1976). Knowing that iodination of tyrosines in the thyroid is essentially related to the structure and availability of thyroglobulin in thyroid tissue it is obvious that abnormalities of thyroid protein metabolism could be expected in thyroid cancer.

1 Abnormal Thyroid Protein Metabolism in Thyroid Cancer

It is generally accepted that proper thyroid hormone synthesis in the thyroid depends on an efficient iodine trapping mechanism – which is obviously blunted in most thyroid cancers – and on the availability of appropriate exons of the thyroglobulin molecule with tyrosines ready for reaction (Monaco, Andreoli 1978). Even as it was mentioned, that sometimes thyroid carcinomas can produce large amounts of thyroid hormones under these preconditions and even release them into the circulation it must be stressed that these cases are rather exceptions to the rule: Usually the malignant development of thyroid cells is accompanied by a variety of alterations in iodine metabolism which are partly due to defective thyroglobulin synthesis (Thomas-Morvan et al. 1974). Thyroglobulin synthesis is a very complex process involving gene transcription, proper structuring of the molecule to avoid too many introns, polyadenylation and mRNA play an essential role. The sugar-chains in the Golgi-apparatus are also important and the terminal sialic acid component in thyroglobulin is essential. Mannose-phosphate may help to target thyroglobulin to lysosomes (Consiglio et al. 1981). Finally thyroglobulin is degraded by proteases. It could therefore be expected that malignant thyroid cells show a wide spectrum of alterations in these complicated reactions. Abnormal iodoproteins are known to be synthesized in thyroid cancer and secreted into the circulation (Van Herle, Uller 1975) sometimes with the characteristics of "albumin". A variety of other abnormal iodoproteins can also occur in the serum of patients with thyroid carcinoma. Several defects of thyroglobulin molecules produced in thyroid carcinomas have been described as well (Robbins 1968) and there is also evidence that a lack of sialo transferase inhibits thyroglobulin secretion in such lesions. In general it can be said – however – that the synthesis and even the release of some kind of thyroglobulin in the circulation is maintained in many thyroid carcinomas, which have lost their capacity to trap iodine and to produce thyroid hormones (Botsch et al. 1979). It is no wonder therefore that iodinated tyrosines are present in such tumors in unusually high amounts, while thyroid hormones can be almost absent. It must nevertheless be stressed, that these phenomena do represent significant changes in thyroid protein metabolism as consequences of the malignant cell transformation and cannot be considered as primary events in the development of thyroid carcinoma. The observation of increased keratin in papillary carcinoma of the thyroid can also be interpreted in this context (Permanetter et al. 1983). Regarding the basic alterations of protein metabolism in malignant cells a considerable amount of information exists (Akimova et al. 1969). Whether the fact, that ^{67}Ga (Fig. 12) seems to bind to

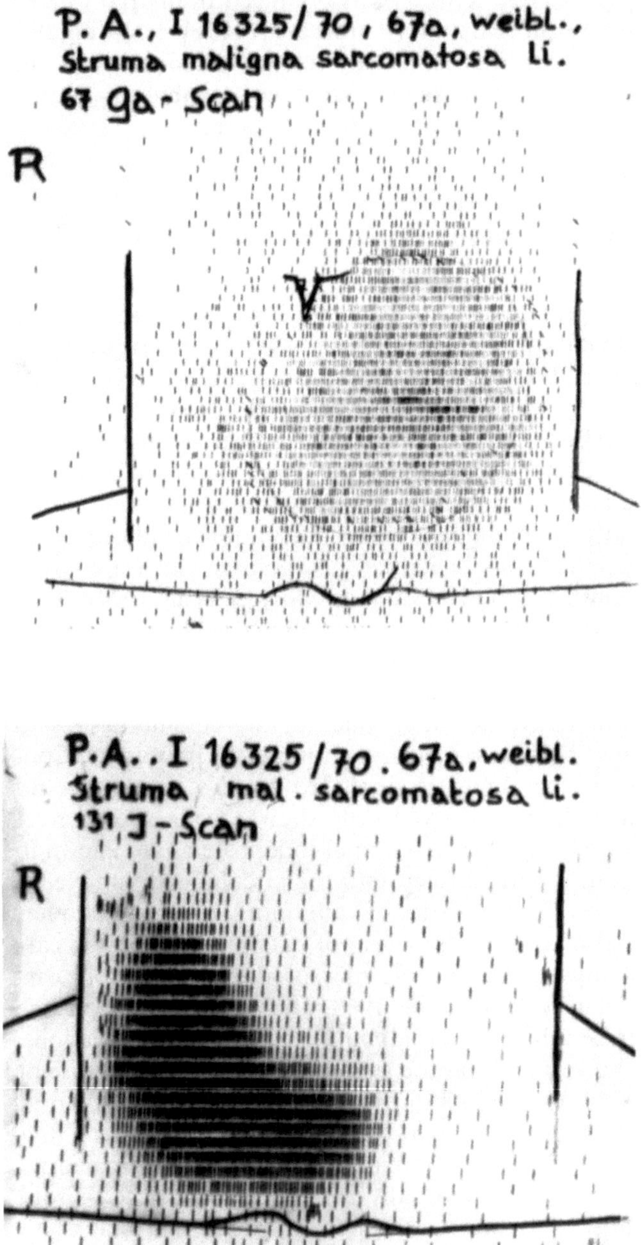

Fig. 12. Intense ^{67}Ga-uptake in thyroid cancer (*above*) in a patient with cold lesion on ^{131}I-scan in left lobe (*below*)

thyroid malignancies is due not only to increased capillary permeability but to specific alterations in the protein metabolism of rapidly proliferating tissues (Gelrud et al. 1974) remains an open question at present. Excessive amounts of lysosomes and sulfhydril bonds and even pH-alterations were observed (Bauer et al. 1975) but all these data on protein metabolism – so far – seem to confirm the hypothesis that such changes do occur in thyroid cancer, that their demonstration can provide additional possibilities for diagnosis, follow-up and – possibly – treatment (see later), but that we cannot correlate them with oncogenesis in the thyroid.

2 TSH, TSH-receptors and cAMP in Thyroid Malignancy

As mentioned above the influence of TSH on the pathophysiology of thyroid cancer and even on it's biological behaviour was noted many years ago (Thomas 1957). It was not only recorded that TSH increased ^{131}I-uptake in thyroid malignancies but also that one could produce thyroid tumors under prolonged TSH-stimulation (Doniach 1963). As the mechanism of TSH action in thyroid cells became known in detail many informations could be obtained concerning the effects of TSH on already existing thyroid cancers:

a) As the TSH-receptor in thyroid cell membranes was defined and it's importance for TSH-action in thyroid tissue became obvious (Tata et al. 1976) it was described also that TSH-receptors do exist in malignant thyroid cells. Their binding capacity, however, varies widely among different tumor types (Kohn et al. 1981). Undifferentiated carcinoma – e.g. – does not contain high affinity TSH-receptors.
b) After binding of TSH to the TSH-receptor the further consequences of TSH-influence on thyroid cell metabolism are mediated by cAMP (DeGroot, Stanbury 1975) and the activity of this interaction is reflected in the activity of the adenylate cyclase system (Goretzki et al. 1983). The message delivered to the thyroid cell by cAMP according to the TSH binding at the receptor site is transmitted by mRNA and would normally include an increase of iodide trapping, a stimulation of energy-providing glucose pathways, of protein synthesis (= also thyroid hormone synthesis) and protease activity (= thyroid hormone release) (Oberdisse et al. 1980). In thyroid cancer, however, it was found that even if TSH-binding to receptors occurs, the metabolic response can be abnormal: There might be no increase in thyroid hormone synthesis in such cells, they might secrete iodoproteins into the circulation which do not contain metabolically active thyroid hormone and peculiar effects on other elements of protein and glucose metabolism may well occur (DeGroot 1983). (Fig. 13). Even if "proper" thyroglobulin synthesis and secretion by thyroid cancer tissue is increased due to TSH, the thyroglobulin produced is still lacking thyroid hormone in many cases, because (see above) it might be unable to synthesize thyroxine and triiodothyronine due to structural abnormalities.

We are sure therefore, that TSH, it's interaction with specific receptors and the transmission of these signals via cAMP do not only represent pathophysio-

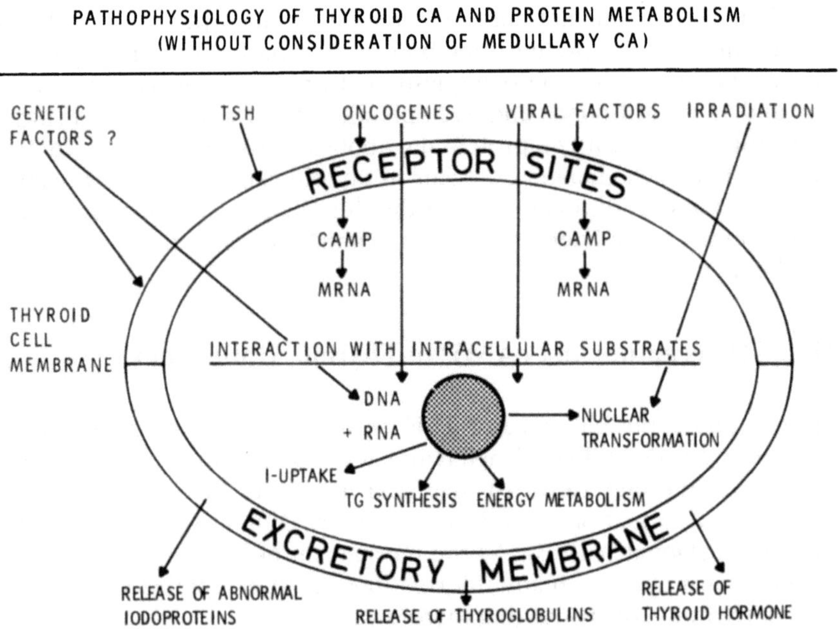

Fig. 13. Pathophysiology and protein metabolism in thyroid cancer (a trial for a model)

logical parameters in thyroic cancer, these phenomena can also modify the behaviour of thyroid cancer and the impact of therapy. Furthermore TSH can perhaps produce thyroid cancer in humans (Furth 1969) and the medical suppression of TSH-secretion can be used to reduce the progression of thyroid malignancies as noted above (Crile 1966). If we could work with sensitive and specific TSH-receptor-assays in thyroid tumors as we do it with estrogen – and/or – progesteron receptor assays in breast cancer (Fasching 1984) a valuable contribution for therapy-planning in thyroid malignancies could be realized. At present, however, the technical difficulties of TSH-receptor-assays in thyroid tissue do not allow the implementation of such programs on a routine basis.

3 Multiple Endocrine Neoplasia with Medullary Thyroid Carcinoma

As mentioned previously the pathophysiological criteria of medullary thyroid carcinoma were recognized rather late and it took a long time until – in such a rare disease – the occurrence of such tumors together with phaeochromocytoma, parathyroid adenomas and neuromas of the GI-tract in families was seen as a proper pathological entity (Williams 1981). At first such cases were considered as a medical curiosity (Sizemore et al. 1977) but with increasing experience it became obvious that 20% of medullary thyroid carcinomas indeed

Table 16. Hereditary multiple endocrine neoplasia [a]

Multiple endocrine neoplasia syndromes (Apudomas)	Old names (S. = syndrome)	Manifestifications (endocrinologically active tumors in . . . .)
Type 1	Wermer -S.	Thyroid, beta-cells pancreas, adrenals, parathyroids
Type 2	Sipple -S.	Thyroid (med. Ca.), phaeochromocytoma, parathyroids
Type 3	Schimke -S.	Thyroid (med. Ca.), phaeochromocytoma, neurinoma (larynx, tongue, buccal mucosa), megacolon

[a] According to "Endokrinologie des Kindes- und Jugendalters", Stolicke H., Springer, Berlin, Heidelberg, New York, 1982

occurred in the genetical framework of what became known as "multiple endocrine neoplasia-syndrome" (MEN) (Sipple 1961, Mannin et al. 1963). Today we can even distinguish between several types of such diseases (Table 16). The clinical pecularities of these syndromes will be described later. Regarding the pathophysiology of such thyroid tumors, however, it was demonstrated, that their ability to produce and secrete calcitonin in excessive amounts was a specific criterium (Williams 1981). Calcitonin is a polypeptide hormone with low molecular weight normally produced by parafollicular C-cells in the thyroid (Wolfe et al. 1973). Elevated blood levels of calcitonin were reported in a variety of non-thyroidal diseases, but it remains unknown at present, whether these findings are due to ectopic production of the hormone or stimulation of the C-cells by other substances (Williams 1981). The physiological role of calcitonin is not yet well understood either: The hormone is obviously an antagonist to parathormone as it can lower blood calcium levels while it decreases calcium release by osteoclastic activity from bone (Verdy et al. 1976), a fact which has been used therapeutically in Paget's disease and other bone disorders (Klein et al. 1971). It's secretion can be stimulated by large doses of calcium i.v. (Parthemore et al. 1974). In cases with borderline serum calcitonin concentrations calcium i.v. has been suggested therefore as a provocative test. The frequent side effects of high calcium doses i.v. such as nausea, flushing etc., however, have made such provocations of calcitonin secretion unpopular. Pentagastrin can also stimulate calcitonin secretion and has been proposed as a substitute for calcium (Wells et al. 1975), although side-effects also occur with this method. Today ethanol – "a good glass of whisky" – drunken rapidly is accepted widely as a reliable provocative test with the least side effects in family screening for MEN (Cohen et al. 1973). It was suggested that alcohol stimulates calcitonin secretion by it's adrenergic effect. Of course we would know nothing or at least much less about the pathophysiology of medullary thyroid carcinoma, if we could not apply sensitive radioimmunoassays to measure calcitonin in blood (Colt et al. 1971) (Table 17). As cells deriving from the ultimobranchial body belong to the APUD (= amine and precursor uptake and decarboxylation) system these syndromes of APUD cell abnormalities are usu-

Table 17. Schematic summary of metabolic abnormalities in thyroid cancer cells

		Adeno-Ca.	Med. Ca.
Membrane	I-uptake	↓	–
	TSH-receptor	±	–
	P-uptake	↑	+
	Tl-uptake	↑	+
Cell	Thyroglobulin synthesis	±	±
	Iodine organification	↓	–
	Thyroid hormone synthesis	↓	–
	DNA-synthesis	↑	+
	Abnormal thyroid proteins	↑	+
	Calcitonin synthesis	–	+

ally reflected by similar pathophysiological criteria. The precise mechanisms by which calcitonin is synthesized in C-cells and their malignant variety is unknown. The frequent symptom of diarrhea could be related to high serotonin and histamine levels in blood mediated by prostaglandins, but it is still not understood completely at present. In MEN – of course – the thyroid pathology can sometime be detected only accidentally, while the hypertensive crises due to a phaechromocytoma or a severe diarrhea are the first reasons for the patients to consult a doctor (see later). It should also be mentioned that medullary thyroid carcinoma does not only produce calcitonin, but that several biologically active substances were detected in elevated concentrations in such tumors: ACTH, somatostatin, β-endorphin, neurotensin and some biogenic amines (ketacalcin) were found in similar lesions (Williams 1981). CEA can also be produced and secreted by medullary thyroid cancer and is therefore even included in follow-up programs of patients with this disease together with calcitonin (Weissel, Höfer 1983). We are left therefore with the fact that medullary thyroid carcinoma is a really peculiar tumor regarding it's pathophysiological behaviour. We do not understand the mechanism and significance of the pathophysiological alterations as yet. It seems certain, however, that the excessive production of calcitonin due to the C-cell origin is a tumor specific feature, while other pathophysiological findings occur as a consequence of a variety of abnormal metabolic patterns in these lesions. In familial MEN great care should also be taken to distinguish in a variety of pathophysiological parameters in blood and urine between those related to medullary thyroid carcinoma and others related to separate endocrinologically active tumors.

Aetiology of Thyroid Cancer

The aetiology of only a few malignancies is known so far: Actinic influences can produce skin cancer, cigarette smoking bronchiogenic carcinoma, Bilharzia infections cancer of the bladder etc. For the majority of other malignancies however, aetiology remains mostly unknown. A number of hypotheses exist involving chemically toxic influences, virus effects and hormonal factors to explain malignant transformations in cell lines. It is widely accepted today that the immune response of the body can modify the development of clinical cancer significantly (Hall et al. 1980). All these considerations naturally apply also to the aetiology of thyroid cancer. Estrogens, pregnancy and lactation do not have any certified significance for the aetiology of thyroid malignancy, it is even a question if these influences can modify the course of the disease (Rosvoll, Winship 1965). A few features, however, are thought to be of special importance regarding thyroid tumors.

1 Iodine Deficiency

In the chapters on epidemiology and pathophysiology of thyroid cancer some facts regarding these old speculations on the influence of iodine deficiency on the pathogenesis of thyroid cancer were already mentioned. Wegelin (Wegelin 1928) was convinced that iodine deficiency promoted the development of thyroid malignancies and it was considered as likely, that thyroid cancer was a frequent transformation of an originally benign thyroid nodule (De Quervain 1941). As such lesions are common in iodine deficient, endemic goiter areas it could be expected, that the incidence of thyroid cancer in such regions would be exceedingly high. A further support for the theory of an important role played by iodine deficiency in the aetiology of thyroid cancer was delivered by the observation that prolonged TSH-stimulation can produce thyroid tumors and increase tumor growth as mentioned earlier: As in the concept of goitrogenesis in general and in iodine deficient endemic goiter countries specifically, TSH is accepted as one significant factor for thyroid growth, it therefore seemed obvious that

a) Iodine deficiency produces increased TSH-secretion via the physiological feedback mechanism,
b) that such increased TSH-influence over a long period would produce thyroid tumors, which

c) by continuation of TSH effects and the inherent life history of thyroid nodules would become malignant.

All this sounded very reasonable. Doubts about this aetiological concept appeared, when it was shown, that high incidences of thyroid cancer exceeding those in endemic goiter areas occurred in regions without iodine deficiency or even with an excessively high iodine intake (see earlier). We have also learned that elevated iodine intake can produce goiter (Gold 1959, Suzuki 1980) and even lymphocytic thyroiditis. As old clinicians used to say: iodine has a "Janus-Head" regarding it's influence on thyroid metabolism and on goiter growth. With the same substance one can treat hyperthyroidism and produce myxedema as well as one can create real thyrotoxicosis. With the same substance one can also shrink existing goiters significantly (Buttfield et al. 1967) or produce thyroid enlargement (Suzuki 1980). The conditions responsible in an individual for the manner in which it's thyroid will react to iodine deficiency or iodine excess are partially known but not perfectly understood at present. Iodine deficiency will decrease thyroid hormone synthesis because even the different adaptation mechanisms of the thyroid do not provide enough iodine for adequate hormone production, while iodine excess can decrease thyroid hormone synthesis by what became known as the Wolff-Chaikoff-effect (Wolff 1969) and reduce thyroid hormone release from the gland (Wartofsky et al. 1970). So finally both conditions will establish a situation, in which due to low levels of circulating thyroid hormone TSH production becomes elevated and thyroid growth can occur. The response of the individual thyroid to abnormal situations in iodine supply seem to be influenced by a variety of immunological phenomena and other factors as discussed later on (Riccabona 1972, Suzuki 1980). It already has been mentioned that iodine deficiency with a goiter endemia can alter the histological picture and clinical course of thyroid cancer. Overall therefore, abnormalities of iodine supply – be it by deficiency or excess – really seem to play a role in the aetiology of thyroid cancer mediated by functional alterations of thyroid hormone metabolism and chronic TSH influence. The significance of such abnormalities, however, in relation to other oncogenic factors can hardly be established precisely at present.

2 Ionizing Radiation

When it became known that children, who had been treated with ionizing radiation for "hyperplasia" of the thymus, tonsils and for hemangiomas on upper chest and neck, developed thyroid cancer in an exceedingly high percentage after a latent period of 10–15 years, the pathogenesis of thyroid cancer due to radiation was clearly defined (Greenspan 1977). Data from populations exposed to atomic blasts completed these reports (Socolow et al. 1963). As a considerable number of publications over the past years (Oberdisse et al. 1980) has shown indeed a direct relationship between the incidence of thyroid cancer and radiation exposure (Fig. 14), the oncogenic effects of ionizing radiation on the

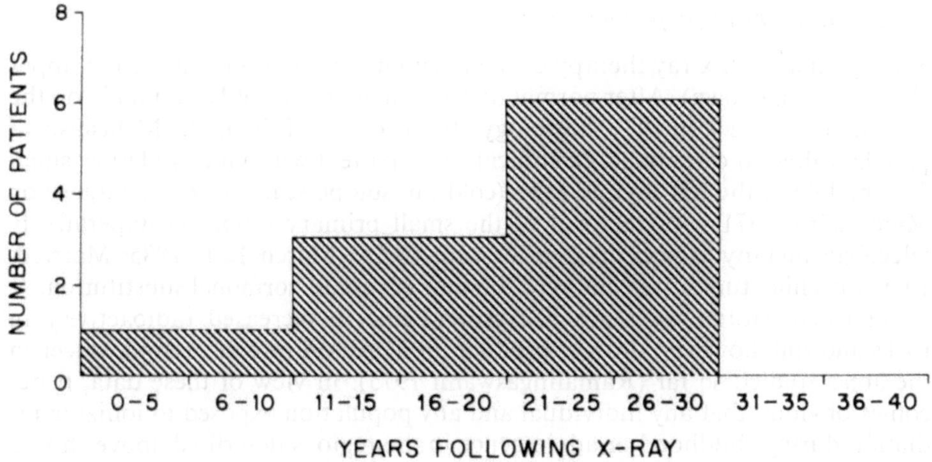

Fig. 14. Influence of ionizing irradiation during childhood on development of thyroid tumors (from DeGroot, Stanbury, 1975)

thyroid gland have attrated increasing interest (De Groot, Reilley 1981). It was reported, that children would respond much more frequently with thyroid malignancy to ionizing radiation than older population groups (Refetoff et al. 1975). This is certainly due to the well-known high sensitivity of juvenile tissues to radiation in relation to the enormous mitosis-rates under these circumstances. One phenomenon in this context remains worthy of further discussion: If a hemangioma or some other lesion in the regions described is irradiated, even with relatively low doses, why does the thyroid develop malignant growth and not any other structures in the surrounding of the irradiated lesion? Even irradiation of the head with a low dose for tinea capitis (thyroid dose 6,5 rad) was reported to provoke thyroid cancer (Lewitus 1983). Where is the dose level which can be considered as responsible for thyroid oncogenesis? How was a proper localization of radiation therapy achieved in each individual case? Regarding thyroid cancers attributed to atomic blasts: How much radiation to the thyroid was delivered by radioactive fallout, and how much by external irradiation? Of course, no linear correlation can be established between Gy to head and neck below 18 years and the incidence of thyroid cancer/1 000 000/year in such studies (De Groot 1983). Largely unknown factors determining local and individual tissue sensitivity to ionizing radiation including DNA-repair-rates etc. are seen every day by radiotherapists and nuclear physicians (Scherer 1976): Some patients tolerate doses of up to 50 Gy to the thyroid without clinical symptoms, while others show intense radiation reactions already with a dose of 20 Gy. As shown later, sequelae of ionizing radiation on neck, thyroid, bone marrow and other organs are known, but they can hardly be defined in each individual case. Overall we know certainly that even rather low doses of ionizing radiation to head, neck, upper chest and thyroid (< 0.05 Gy) can produce thyroid cancer with a latent period of 10–20 years in 8% of irradiated people.

Case M.I., 59.09.12.56, female, 15 years

Shortly after birth x-ray therapy of hemangioma on the right side of the upper chest (dose unknown). After normal development growth of lymph node on the left side of the neck in 1971. Histology after excision of the node: Metastasis of papillary thyroid carcinoma. In clinical exam patient without complaints, small firm nodule in the left thyroid lobe (cold on isotope scan). Radical surgery on March 23rd, 1971 with removal of the small primary lesion. Postoperatively telecobalt therapy to neck in 2 series with 60 Gy. March 10th, 1985: Married, 1 healthy child, tumor free, euthyroid under adequate hormonal substitution.

Elevated natural radiation background due to increased radioactivity in rocks and soil, however, did not produce an increased rate of thyroid cancer in the areas studied so far (Ramalingaswami 1975). In view of these data, it becomes obvious, that any individual and any population exposed to ionizing radiation during childhood or adolescence in the regions described above should be observed closely for 2 decades regarding the growth of thyroid tumors (De Groot, Reilley 1981). The oncogenic effect of such influences is perhaps the best defined factor concerning the aetiology of thyroid cancer. Still it does not cover the pathogenesis of the vast majority of thyroid cancer cases. The obvious question comes up, why the widespread use of ^{131}I for therapy of benign thyroid disease – even when applied during childhood or adolescence (Sheline et al. 1959) – so far could not be connected with the development of thyroid cancer according to large-scale follow-up studies. Actually it is assumed, that low radiation doses as described in other radiation exposures can enhance malignant transformation in tissue, while the high doses delivered by ^{131}I-therapy actually "kill" thyroid cells without potential for further malignant development (Emrich 1979). The general informations of radiobiology (Streffet 1969) can therefore be applied also to the thyroid gland: Low doses can have a disproportional oncogenic effect especially in a young population, while high doses can kill cancer and do not represent an increased cancer risk regarding the thyroid gland per se.

3 Other Environmental Factors

For us the most striking observation in this regard was the fact, that we actually know 4 couples with thyroid cancer (see Table 18). Besides the reports on increased thyroid cancer incidence in families, which might partly be attributed to genetic factors in the pathogenesis of thyroid malignancy, the statistically significant elevation of thyroid cancer among couples living together could be attributed to oncogenic influences on the thyroid in the "habitat" of these patients (Riccabona et al. 1983). We studied water, natural radiation exposure and soil in the localities where our patients lived with a variety of chemical, physical and bacteriological criteria. No evidence, however, could be produced regarding carcinogens in the environment or elevated natural radiation doses in these cases. The slightly abnormal pattern of Neopterin excretion could be interpreted as a sign either of disturbed immunological situations or of virus in-

Table 18a. Environmental data in homes of couples with thyroid Ca.

	Water			Urine		TLD readings
	Quality	$^{14}C/^{3}H/^{90}Sr$	I	$^{14}C/^{3}H/^{90}Sr$	μg I/g creat ($\bar{x}$)	
Fam. M. J.	Quality poor (E. coli!)	Ø	< 3 μg/l	Ø	109	Max. 21 mr above background (well!)
Fam. M. A.	Good	Ø	< 3 μg/l	Ø	78	Background

Table 18b. Neopterin in 24 hr-urines of families in which both parents had thyroid Ca. (μmol/l, upper normal level < 250 μmol/mol creatinine)

	$\bar{x}$	Remarks
Fam. M. J./M. J. (n = 3)	166	1 out of 3 elevated (254)
Fam. M. A./M. A. (n = 5)	552	3 out of 5 elevated (277, 912, 1158)
Total	408	4 out of 8 elevated

fections (Vecchio et al. 1981). Data exist showing, that retroviruses – especially of the murine sarcoma type – can produce thyroid cell transformations in cell cultures by recombining their RNA with a host cell genoma and/or leukemia virus oncogens. The results of these studies were usually anaplastic thyroid cancers. The suggestion that virus infections could therefore produce malignant developments in epithelial cells – which might also produce a specific DNA-configuration with a potential for malignant growth – remains a very interesting hypothesis for the aetiology of thyroid cancer, if seen together with our clinical observations. It must be mentioned, however, that such developments were so far only observed in cell cultures of animal thyroids and that we lack any evidence of oncogenic virus infections in human thyroids (Oberdisse et al. 1980). As even in the animal model in tumor cells produced by virus infections no viruses or virus particles could be identified it will be very difficult to assess the oncogenic effects of virus infections in human thyroids "in vivo". In the author's personal opinion the aetiology of thyroid cancers by virus infections would seem quite acceptable in many cases: We know little villages with a series of thyroid cancer cases although – of course – the statistical impact of these observations can hardly be assessed due do the rarity of this disease.

Other carcinogenic substances in water, soil and food as well as in occupational activities do not involve an increased risk of thyroid cancer according to available data (Alderson 1980).

It would be up to microbiologists to develop methods for the screening of virus influences on oncogenesis in the human thyroid gland and the results of such studies would probably open a new dimension to our understanding of the aetiology of thyroid cancer. Recently several oncogens have been demonstrated in thyroid tissue but their role seems uncertain so far as it was suggested that they might transfer a slowly growing tumor in an aggressive one.

4 Genetic Factors

Here again our own observations were important to conceive the possible impact of genetically transmitted oncogenesis in thyroid gland: It seems clear, that families exist (see Fig. 4), in which even as the family members were living far apart thyroid cancer occurs in an exceedingly high incidence (Riccabona 1983). (Another family with 3 follicular carcinomas in 1 generation has been registered recently). As mentioned previously, medullary thyroid carcinoma in the context of a familiar MEN-syndrome is responsible for $\sim$20% of medullary thyroid cancers and these tumors are transmitted by genetical codes in a dominant way (Williams 1981). In such cases, the primary effect of the specific genetic code seems to produce a hyperplasia of C-cells originating from the ultimobranchial body. It remains unknown at present, why those hyperplastic C-cells undergo malignant transformation in some individuals and not in others. If such a genetic aberration would always induce medullary thyroid carcinoma the afflicted family would be extinct by now considering the frequently insufficient treatment models in earlier times. It therefore seems clear, that genes determine the hyperplasia of C-cells but not their malignant transformation.

It should be also considered, that genetic abnormalities involving defects in thyroid hormonogenesis are combined with a chronically increased TSH-stimulation of the thyroid (Doniach 1963). In view of what has been said above it is therefore not surprising that several cases in twins were reported (Winship, Rosvoll 1961). In such patients, however, the genetically conditioned oncogenesis in the thyroid glands obviously is not related to direct oncogenic gene-effects on thyroid cells but rather to chronically increased TSH-stimulation due to genetic abnormalities which then can produce malignant growth in thyroid cells (Furth 1969).

Even as genetic influences therefore do play a role in the aetiology of various forms of thyroid cancer they certainly can "explain" only a relatively small number of such tumors. It seems desirable that centers dealing with the disease would regularly check pedigrees and family connections of relevant patients. An appropriate information in sufficient numbers concerning this problem would certainly provide a valuable knowledge on aetiology of thyroid cancer and could probably promote some kind of genetic counseling or screening programs in afflicted families.

5 Immunological Factors

It has been known for years that the incidence of malignant lymphomas is elevated in Hashimoto's thyroiditis (Burke et al. 1977). Some forms of thyroid carcinoma (especially sclerosing papillary microcarcinoma Graham) were observed frequently in thyroid glands afflicted by Graves' Disease with lymphocytic infiltration (Graham 1925). It would seem therefore, that autoimmunologically conditioned thyroid diseases include an elevated risk of thyroid cancer (Goudie 1969). The current concepts of immunology regarding the thyroid gland and the host response to malignant growth are very general (Frati 1981).

A number of questions arise in this regard:

a) Do thyroid autoantibodies as observed in Hashimoto's Disease (Bastenie, Ermans 1972) stimulate the growth of malignant cells in the thyroid?
b) Do thyroid-growth-stimulating-autoantibodies have the potential not only to stimulate the growth of goiters but can they specifically mediate malignant transformation in thyroid cells?
c) Do lymphocytic infiltrations around or in thyroid carcinomas represent an important defense mechanism of the host organism against tumor progression?

Several reports stated, that prognosis of thyroid cancer – especially of papillary thyroid carcinoma – would correlate well with the degree of lymphocytic infiltration in such lesions, as with the increasing presence of lymphocytes, prognosis became better. Whether all these immunological aspects of the aetiology of thyroid cancer are connected with other aetiological factors cannot be answered at present. Of course we have mentioned the correlation of lymphocytic thyroiditis and iodine excess in nutrition, and it is difficult to distinguish in families which thyroid cancer cases are related to genetic influences, to viral infections or to genetically determined alterations in the immune system. There seems to be a good chance that a variety of oncogenic factors can combine and finally produce "thyroid cancer" and the immune system should not be forgotten in research and clinical judgement.

6 Conclusions

Overall a variety of aetiological factors relevant for thyroid cancer could be defined during the past years. So far it seems that these known aetiological influences (Table 19) can explain only a relatively small proportion of thyroid cancer cases with adequate certainty. As in cancer in general the aetiology of thyroid cancer in detail remains unknown in the majority of cases. It is clear, that in view of all the missing information research on all aspects of cancer aetiology and especially on molecular transformations in thyroid cells resulting in malignant growth would be welcome in the whole medical community.

Table 19. Aetiological factors in thyroid Ca.

Factor's significance	Characterization	Responsible for x % of thyroid Ca.
Well-defined	Radiation to neck and upper chest	1%
	Chronic TSH-stimulation of existing goiter	2%
	Hashimoto's thyroiditis	0.5%
	Genetic influences	~ 1%
Possibly important	Viral infections "oncogenes"	~ 10% (?)
Unclear	Other environmental factors?	~ 84.5% (?)
	Iodine excess?	
	Iodine deficiency?	

References

Abdel-Razzak M, Christie M (1979) Thyroid carcinoma in an autonomously functioning nodule. J Nucl Med 20:1001

Ackerman NB, Marvin JF (1963) The use of radioactive phosphorus in the diagnosis of thyroid cancer. Radiology 77:793

Akimova RN, Ganina KP, Zotikov LA, Lulic GI (1969) Results of a biochemical, histochemical and ultrastructural study of the thyroid gland in the process of experimental cancerogenesis. In: Hedinger Chr (ed) Thyroid Cancer. Springer, Berlin, p 149

Alderson MR (1980) Epidemiology. In: Duncan W (ed) Thyroid Cancer. Springer, Berlin Heidelberg New York, p 9

Andreoli M, Monaco F, Robbins J (1981) Advances in thyroid neoplasia. Field Educational Italia, Roma

Bastenie PA, Ermans AM (1972) Thyroiditis and thyroid function. Pergamon Press, Oxford

Bauer H, Glatzl J, Falkensammer M, Platzer S, Riccabona G (1973) Epidemiologische Besonderheiten zweier benachbarter Kropfgebiete, wovon in einem seit 10 Jahren eine Jodprophylaxe läuft. Acta endocrinol. (Kbh) Suppl 179, p 21

Bauer H, Riccabona G, Salzer GM, Hagleitner E, Lederer B, Glasowski P (1975) Die Ga-67-Speicherung in Malignomen in vitro und ihre Bedeutung für die Klinik. In: Nuklearmedizin. Medico, Berlin, p 832

Baylin SB, Garm DS, Hsu SH (1976) Clonal origin of inherited medullary thyroid carcinoma and phaechromocytoma. Science 193:321

Becker HD, Röher HD, Peitsch W, Wahl RA (1984) Chirurgie der malignen Struma. In: Maligne Schilddrüsentumoren. Springer, Berlin Heidelberg New York Tokyo

Black RM, Woolner LB, Blackburn CM (1953) The uptake of radioactive iodine by carcinoma of the thyroid gland: a study of 128 cases. J Clin Endocrinol 13:1378

Botsch H, Schulz E, Lochner B (1979) Serumthyreoglobulinbestimmung zur Verlaufskontrolle bei Schilddrüsencarcinom-Patienten. Dtsch Med Wschr 104:1072

Breitner B (1925) Das Karzinom der Schilddrüse. Wien med Wschr 1:1

Breitner B, Just E (1924) Die Struma maligna. Mittlg Grenzgeb Med u. Chir, p 262

Burke JS, Butler JJ, Fuller LM (1977) Malignant lymphomas of the thyroid. Cancer 39:1587

Buttfield IH, Hetzel BS (1967) Endemic goiter in Eastern New Guinea with special reference of the use of iodized oil in prophylaxis and treatment. Bull WHO 36:243

Caillou B, Talbot M, Schlumberger M, Rougier Ph, Bellet D, Travagli JP (1983) Usefulness of new methodological and conceptual approaches in thyroid carcinoma. Acta endocrinol (Kbh) Suppl 252, p 29

Caviedes R, Stanbury JB (1976) Studies on a cell-line from a rat thyroid tumor in continous culture. Endocrinology 99:548

Chiovato L, van den Gaag RD, Hanafusa T, Drexhage HA, Doniach D, Bottazzo GF (1984) The growing importance of receptor antibodies in thyroidology. In: Schatz H, Doniach D (ed) Autoimmunity in thyroid disorders. Thieme-Stratton, New York Stuttgart, p 65

Clark RL, Hill CS, White EC (1969) Results of treatment of thyroid cancer by radical surgery. In: Hedinger ChrE (ed) Thyroid Cancer. Springer, Berlin

Clute C, Warren L (1935) The prognosis of thyroid cancer. Surg Gynec Obstet 60:861

Cohen SL, Graham-Smith D, MacIntyre F, Walker JG (1973) Alcohol-stimulated calcitonin release in medullary carcinoma of the thyroid. Lancet II/1172

Colt EWD, Miles LEM, Becker KL, Shaw NI (1971) A sensitive new immunoassay for calcitonin employing labeled antibody. J Clin Endocrinol 32:285

Consiglio E, Kohn LD, Salvatore G, Slufrin S, Cavallo R, Formisano S (1981) Mannose phosphate as a specific signal in the lysosomal biodegradation of thyroglobulin. In: Andreoli M, Monaco F, Robbins J (ed) Advances in thyroid neoplasia. Field Educational Italia, Roma, p 61

Crile G jr (1966) Endocrine dependency of papillary carcinomas of the thyroid. J.A.M.A. 195:721

Dargent M (1948) Thyroidectomy with block dissection of the neck for carcinoma of the thyroid gland. Lancet, p 721

DeGroot LJ (1983) Etiology and pathophysiology of thyroid carcinoma. Acta endocrinol (Kbh), Suppl 252, p 37

DeGroot LJ, Stanbury JB (1975) The thyroid and it's diseases. Wiley & Sons, New York London Sidney Toronto

DeGroot LJ, Reilley M (1981) Radiation-associated thyroid neoplasia. In: Andreoli M et al. (ed) Advances in thyroid neoplasia. Field Educational Italia, Roma, p 149

Denies H, Grapow H, Westendorf W (1958) Grundriß der Medizin der alten Ägypter. Bd. IV, 1. Teil, Berlin, p 223

DeQuervain F (1941) Die Struma maligna. Enke, Stuttgart

Dinsmore RS, Dempsey WS, Hazard JB (1949) Lymphosarcoma of the thyroid. J Clin Endocrinol 9:1043

Dinstl K, Keminger K (1967) Experimentelle Untersuchungen über das metastasierende Schilddrüsenadenom. Klin Med 22:262

Doniach I (1963) Aetiological considerations in thyroid carcinoma. In: The thyroid and it's diseases. Lippincott, Philadelphia, p 106

Edmonds CJ, Hayes S, Kermode JC, Thompson BD (1977) Measurement of serum TSH and thyroid hormones in the management of treatment of thyroid carcinoma with radioiodine. Br J Radiol, 50:799

Ekholm R (1964) Thyroid gland. In: Kurtz SM (ed) Electron microscopic anatomy. Academic Press, New York, p 221

Ellenberg AH, Goldman L, Gordan GS, Lindsay S (1962) Thyroid carcinoma in patients with hyperparathyroidism. Surgery 51:708

Emrich D (1979) Nuklearmedizin – Funktionsdiagnostik und Therapie. Thieme, Stuttgart

Fasching W (1984) Manual der chirurgischen Krebstherapie. Facultas, Wien

Fish J, Moore RM (1963) Ectopic thyroid tissue and ectopic thyroid carcinoma. Ann Surg 157:212

Franssila K (1971) Value of histological classification of thyroid cancer. Acta pathol microbiol Scand (Sect A), Suppl 225

Frati L (1981) Experimental bases of immunochemotherapy of tumors. In: Advances in thyroid neoplasia. Field Educational Italia, Roma, p 275

Fukunaga FH, Lockett JL (1971) Thyroid carcinoma in the Japanese in Hawaii. Arch Pathol 92:6

Furth J (1969) Concepts of thyroidal carcinogenesis: Interpretation of events. Needed research. In: Hedinger ChrE (ed) Thyroid Cancer. Springer, Berlin, p 171

Galvan G (1983) The value of the aspiration cytology for the diagnosis of thyroid malignancies. Acta Endocrinol (Kbh), Suppl 252, p 55

Gebrud LG, Arseneau JC, Milder MS, Kramer RJ, Swann SJ, Canellos GP, Johnston GS (1974) Kinetics of Gallium-67 incorporation into inflammatory lesions: experimental and clinical studies. J Lab Clin Med 83:489

Gold E (1959) Iodide induced goiter. Surgery 45:424

Goretzki PE, Roeher HD, Gerand PL, Nissenson RA, Clark OH (1983) TSH receptors in benign and malignant thyroid neoplasms. Acta Endocrinol (Kbh), Suppl 252, p 39

Goudie RB (1968) Immune relationships of thyroid tumors. In: Young S, Inman DR (ed) Thyroid neoplasia. Academic Press, London, p 363

Graham A (1925) Malignant tumors of the thyroid, epithelial types. Ann Surg 81:30

Greenspan FS (1977) Radiation exposure and thyroid cancer. J Amer med Ass 237:2089

Hakama M (1969) Different world thyroid cancer rates. In: Hedinger ChrE (ed) Thyroid Cancer. Springer, Berlin Heidelberg New York, p 66

Hall R, Ross M, Reng CS, Rees-Smith B (1980) Immunological aspects of thyroid cancer. In: Duncan W (ed) Thyroid Cancer. Springer, Berlin Heidelberg New York, p 56

Hazard JB, Crile G jr, Dempsey WS (1949) Non encapsulated sclerosing tumors of the thyroid. J Clin Endocrinol Metab 9:1216

Hedinger ChrE (1983) Pathology of thyroid cancer. Acta Endocrinol (Kbh), Suppl 252, 102:25

Hedinger ChrE, Sobin LH (1974) Histological typing of thyroid tumors. In: International classification of tumors. WHO Nr. 11, Geneva

Heimann R, Vanninense A, deSloover C, Dor P (1978) Malignant lymphomas and undifferentiated small cell carcinoma of the thyroid: a clinicopathological review in the light of the Kiel classification for malignant lymphomas. Histopathology 2:201

Hempelmann LH, Hall WJ, Phillips M, Cooper RA, Ames WR (1975) Neoplasms in persons treated with x-rays in infancy: fourth survey in 20 years. J Natl Cancer Inst 55:519

Hofstädter F (1983) Electron microscope and cytochemical studies: differentiation of follicular and anaplastic thyroid carcinoma. Acta Endocrinol (Kbh), Suppl 252, p 32

Horst W (1961) Klinische Radiojoddiagnostik der Schilddrüsenerkrankungen. In: Künstliche radioaktive Isotope in Physiologie, Diagnostik und Therapie. Bd 2, Springer, Berlin Göttingen Heidelberg, p 886

Horst W, Heuwieser H (1957) Radiopapierchromatographische Untersuchungen zur Frage der endokrinen Leistung des Schilddrüsencarcinoms als Basis für die Radiojodtherapie. Strahlenther 102:379

Huber P, Riccabona G (1967) Diagnostik und Therapie der Schilddrüsenerkrankungen vom Gesichtspunkt des Chirurgen aus. In: Klinische Chirurgie für die Praxis. Erg.Bd, Thieme, Stuttgart

Huber P, Riccabona G (1969) Die Lebensaussichten der malignen Strumen. Wien med Wschr 119:143

Jao W, Gould VE (1975) Ultrastructure of anaplastic carcinoma of the thyroid. Cancer 35:1280

Ibanez ML, Russell WO, Albores-Saavedra J, Lampertico P, White EC, Clark RL (1966) Thyroid carcinoma – biologic behaviour and mortality. Cancer 19:1039

Klein E, Reinwein D (1978) Klinische Endokrinologie. Schattauer, Stuttgart New York

Klinck GH (1969) Hemangioendothelioma and sarcoma of the thyroid. UICC Monogr Series, Springer, Berlin Heidelberg New York, p 60

Kocher A (1924) Die malignen Tumoren der Schilddrüse. In: Zweifel & Payr: Die Klinik der bösartigen Geschwülste. Leipzig, Vol 1

Kohn LD, Meldolesi MF, Aloj SM, Vitti P, Valente WA, Laccetti P, Cohen JL, Dianzani U, Grollmann EF (1981) A molecular model of the thyrotropin receptor: experimental and human thyroid tumors with relevant defects. In: Advances in thyroid neoplasia. Field Educational Italia, Roma, p 23

Kurihara et al (1984) Cancer mortality statistics in the world, part I: Malignant neoplasm of thyroid gland. WHO, p. 32

Ladurner D, Hofstädter F, Riccabona G (1979) Schilddrüsenchirurgie vor und nach Einführung der Kropfprophylaxe. Kongr Ber Österr Ges f Chir, Demeter, München

Ladurner D, Seeber G (1984) Das follikuläre Schilddrüsenkarzinom. Schweiz med Wschr 114:1087

Lahey FH, Ficarra BJ (1946) Lateral aberrant thyroid gland. Surg Gyn obstet 82:705

Lewitus Z (1983) Thyroid carcinoma in Israel. Acta Endocrinol (Kbh), Suppl 252, p 15

Lindsay S (1960) Carcinoma of the thyroid gland. Thomas, Springfield/Ill., USA

Major RH (1954) A history of medicine. Springfield

Mannin PC, Molnar GD, Black BM, Priestley JT, Woolner LB (1963) Phaeochromocytoma, hyperparathyroidism and thyroid carcinoma occuring coincidently. New Eng J Med 268:68

Mayberger HW (1959) Adenocarcinoma of thyroid origin in a benign cystic teratoma. Amer J Obstet Gynec 78:817

Monaco F, Andreoli M (1978) Hormonogenetic errors in thyroid tumor. J Endocrinol Invest 1:373

Niepomenisze H, Altschuler N, Korob MH, Degrossi OJ (1969) Iodide peroxydase activity in human thyroid. Acta Endocrinol (Kbh) 62:193

Oberdisse K, Klein E, Reinwein D (1980) Die Krankheiten der Schilddrüse. Thieme, Stuttgart New York

Österr Bds Ges Bl 1963

Palmieri B (1981) Cryoprint system for intraoperative diagnosis in thyroid surgery: a perspective. In: Andreoli M, Monaco F, Robbins J (ed) Advances in thyroid neoplasia. Field Educational Italia, Roma, p 325

Parthemore JG, Bronzert D, Roberts G, Deftos LJ (1974) A short calcium infusion in the diagnosis of medullary thyroid carcinoma. J Clin Endocrinol 39:108

Patton JA, Hallifield JW, Brill AB, Lee GS, Patton DD (1976) Differentiation between malignant and benign solitary thyroid nodules by fluorescent scanning. J Nucl Med 17:17

Pemberton J (1939) Malignant lesions of the thyroid gland: review of 774 cases. Surg Gynec Obstet 69:417

Permanetter W, Nathrath WBJ, Löhrs U, Gärtner R (1983) Immunohistochemical studies of keratin and thyroglobulin in thyroid tumors. Acta Endocrinol (Kbh), Suppl 252, p 40

Pfaltz M, Hedinger ChrE, Mühlethaler JP (1983) Mixed medullary and follicular carcinoma of the thyroid. Virchow's Arch path Anat 400:53

Platzer S, Groebner P, Hausen A, Obendorf L, Riccabona G (1980) Schilddrüsenproteine in endemischen Strumen und ihre Beziehung zur intrathyreoidalen Schilddrüsenhormonkonzentration. Wien klin Wschr 92:88

Pochin EE, Thompson B (1969) Metabolic activity of tumor tissue. In: Hedinger ChrE (ed) Thyroid Cancer. Springer, Berlin Heidelberg New York, p 194

Raith L, Locher D, Engelhart D, Karl HJ (1970) Thyreotoxische Krise bei Schilddrüsenmalignomen. Internist 11:146

Ramalingaswami V (1975) Personal comm.

Refetoff S, Harrison JR, Karanfilski BT, Kaplan EL, DeGroot LJ, Bekerman C (1975) Continuing occurrence of thyroid carcinoma after irradiation to the neck in infancy and childhood. N Engl J Med 292:171

Riccabona G (1972) Die endemische Struma. Urban & Schwarzenberg, München Berlin Wien

Riccabona G (1982) Epidemiologie der Struma maligna. Schweiz med Rundschau 71:523

Riccabona G, Oberladstätter M, Fill H, Zechmann W, Fuchs D, Jenewein I (1983) Incidence of thyroid cancer in families: some case reports. Acta Endocrinol (Kbh), Suppl 252, p 19

Robbins J (1968) Abnormal thyroglobulin in experimental rat thyroid tumor. In: Young S, Iman DR (ed) Thyroid Neoplasia. Academic Press, New York, p 405

Rosvoll RV, Winship T (1965) Thyroid carcinoma and pregnancy. Surg Gynec Obstet 121:1039

Russel MA, Gilbert EF, Jaeschke WF (1975) Prognostic features of thyroid cancer

Schauer A (1984) Pathogenese and pathologische Anatomie. In: Becker HD, Heinze HG (ed) Maligne Schilddrüsentumoren. Springer, Berlin Heidelberg New York Tokyo, p 2

Scherer E (1976) Strahlentherapie. Springer, Berlin Heidelberg New York

Schottenfeld D, Berg JW (1971) Incidence of multiple primary cancers. IV.: Cancers of the female breast and genital organs. J Natl Cancer Inst 46:161

Schottenfeld D, Gershman St (1977) Epidemiology of thyroid cancer, part 2. Clin Bull 7:98

Schroeder S, Boecker W, Huesselmann H, Dralle H (1984) Adenolipoma (thyrolipoma) of the thyroid gland: report of 2 cases and review of literature. Virchow's Arch Pathol Anat 404:99

Shapiro SJ, Friedman NB, Perzik SL, Catz B (1970) Incidence of thyroid cancer in Graves' disease. Cancer 26:1261

Sheline GE, Lindsay S, Bell HG (1959) Occurrence of thyroid nodules in children following therapy with radioactive iodine for hyperthyroidism. J Clin Endocrinol 19:127

Shimaoka K, Sokal JE, Pickren JW (1962) Metastatic neoplasms in the thyroid gland. Cancer 15:557

Sipple JH (1961) The association of phaeochromocytoma with carcinoma of the thyroid gland. Amer J Med 31:163

Sizemore GW, Carney JA, Heath H (1977) Epidemiology of medullary carcinoma of the thyroid gland: A 5-year experience. Surg Clin Am 57:633

Socolow EL, Hashizuma A, Neriishi S, Niitani R (1963) Thyroid carcinoma in man after exposure to ionizing radiation. New Engl J Med 268:406

Stanbury JB, Hedge AN (1950) A study of a family of goitrous cretins. J Clin Endocrinol 10:1471
Stanburg JB, Hetzel BS (1980) Endemic goiter and endemic cretinism. Wiley & Sons, New York Toronto Chichester Brisbane
Streffer C (1969) Strahlen-Biochemie. Springer, Berlin Heidelberg New York
Sturgeon CT, Davis FE, Catz B, Petit D, Starr P (1953) Treatment of thyroid cancer metastases with TSH and ^{131}I during thyroid hormone medication. J Clin Endocrinol 13:1391
Suzuki H (1980) Etiology of endemic goiter and iodide excess. In: Stanbury JB, Hetzel BS (ed) Endemic goiter and endemic cretinism. Wiley & Sons, New York Chichester Brisbane Toronto, p 237
Tata RL, Winaud RJ, Kohn LD (1976) Solubilization and partial purification of the thyrotropin receptor. In: Robbins J, Braverman L (ed) Thyroid research. International Congress Series Nr. 378. Excerpta Medica, Amsterdam, p 57
Thaler W, Riccabona G, Riedler L, Schmid K (1986) Zum malignen Haemangioendotheliom der Schilddrüse. Chirurg 57:397
Thomas CG (1957) Hormonal treatment of thyroid cancer. J Clin Endocrinol Metab 17:232
Thomas-Morvan C, Nataf B, Tubiana M (1974) Thyroid proteins and hormone synthesis in human thyroid cancer. Acta Endocrinol (Kbh) 76:651
Urban K (1938) Die Chirurgie des Kropfes. Deuticke, Leipzig Wien
Van Herle AJ, Uller RP (1975) Elevated serum thyroglobulin. J Clin Invest 56:272
Verdy M, Beaulieu R, Demars L, Sturdridge WC, Thomas P, Kumar MA (1971) Plasma calcitonin activity in a patient with medullary thyroid carcinoma and her children with osteoporosis. J Clin Endocrinol 32:216
Waldhart B (1969) Die Schilddrüse. In: Doerr W, Seifert G, Uehlinger E (ed) Spezielle pathologische Anatomie. Springer, Berlin, Vol 4, p 321
Waldhart B (1963) Der Gestaltwandel der Struma maligna mit Bezug auf die Jodprophylaxe des Kropfes. Schweiz med Wschr 93:809
Walther HE (1948) Krebsmetastasen. Schwabe, Basel
Ward R (1949) When is malignant goiter malignant? J Clin Endocrinol 9:1031
Wartofsky C, Ransil BJ, Ingbar SH (1970) Inhibition by iodide of the release of thyroxine from the glands of patients with thyrotoxicosis. J Clin Invest 49:78
Wegelin C (1926) Schilddrüse. In: Lubarsch O, Henke F, Rossle R, Uehlinger E (ed) Spezielle pathologische Anatomie und Histologie. Springer, Berlin, Vol VIII
Wegelin C (1928) Malignant disease of the thyroid gland and its relation to goiter in man and animals. Cancer Rev 3:297
Weinstein JB, Kitchin FD (1971) Genetic factors in thyroid diseases. In: Werner SC, Ingbar SH (ed) The thyroid. Harper & Row, New York
Weissel M, Höfer R (1983) Carcinoembryonic antigen (CEA) in thyroid cancer. Acta Endocrinol (Kbh), Suppl 252, p 60
Wells SA, Ontjes DA, Cooper CW, Hennessy JT, Ellis GJ, McPherson HT, Sabiston DC (1975) The early diagnosis of medullary carcinoma of the thyroid gland in patients with multiple endocrine neoplasia. Ann Surg 182:360
Williams ED (1979) Medullary carcinoma of the thyroid. In: DeGroot LJ (ed) Endocrinology. Grune & Stratton, New York, Vol 2, p 777
Williams ED (1981) C-cells and C-cell tumors in animals and man. In: Andreoli A, Monaco F, Robbins J (ed) Advances in thyroid neoplasia. Field Educational Italia, Roma, p 123
Williams ED, Doniach I, Bjarnason O, Michie W (1977) Thyroid cancer in an iodide rich area. Cancer 39:215
Williams ED (1980) Pathology and natural history. In: Duncan W (ed) Thyroid cancer. Springer, Berlin Heidelberg New York, p 47
Winand RJ, Kohn LD (1975) Thyrotropin effects on thyroid cells in culture: effects of trypsin on the thyrotropin receptor and on thyrotropin-mediated cyclic 3′:5′-AMP changes. J Biol Chem 250:6534
Winship T, Roscoll RV (1961) Childhood thyroid carcinoma. Cancer 14:734
Wolfe HJ, Melvin KEW, Cervi-Skinner SJ, Al Saadi AA, Juliar JF, Jackson CE, Tashjian AH (1973) C-cell hyperplasia preceding medullary thyroid carcinoma. N Engl J Med 289:437
Wolff J (1969) Iodide goiter and the pharmacological effects of excess iodide. Am J Med 47:101

B
Clinical Picture, Diagnosis, Therapy and Follow-up

Clinical Features

1 Relevant Symptoms

It is natural, that in a tumor with such a variety of histological and pathophysiological properties also clinical symptoms vary considerably (Schwarz, Scriba 1969).

Type 1:

The classical picture of thyroid cancer is usually seen in anaplastic carcinomas and/or sarcomas and is – as mentioned previously – fortunately a rare story: It has been described many times (Huber 1956), but for the sake of completeness it should briefly be mentioned once more: rapid growth of a thyroid mass, increasing dyspnoea, dysphagia, sometimes pain with retroauricular extension to the head and/or to the shoulder and arm, hoarseness, weakness. All these symptoms can develop rapidly over a period of a few weeks, in other cases the evolution of the disease is slower and can take months. Anyway the correct diagnosis can usually be made on the basis of the history alone.

Type 2:

Patients with better differentiated thyroid tumors usually report growth of a single nodule in the neck over a period of several months. Sometimes the nodule is tender and firm, so that in developed countries with a widespread fear of malignancy and without endemic goiter problems, these – otherwise symptomless patients – seek medical consultation. Sometimes thyroid hormone therapy was given for months but the nodule did not respond or even grew larger.

Type 3:

The primary lesion only becomes apparent due to complaints from metastases. These may be indolent lymph-node swellings in the neck (naturally without response to frequently prescribed antibiotic medication), an excision reveals that they are lymph node metastases of thyroid cancer, no other complaints exist (Horn 1955). On the other hand patients see their doctors because of "rheumatic" pains in spine or legs, because of shortness of breath with bloody sputum or because of a lump on the scalp which they notice when they are combing their hair. Sometimes (10–20%) they will say that they had thyroid surgery years ago (no histology available), chest or bone films will reveal osteolytic

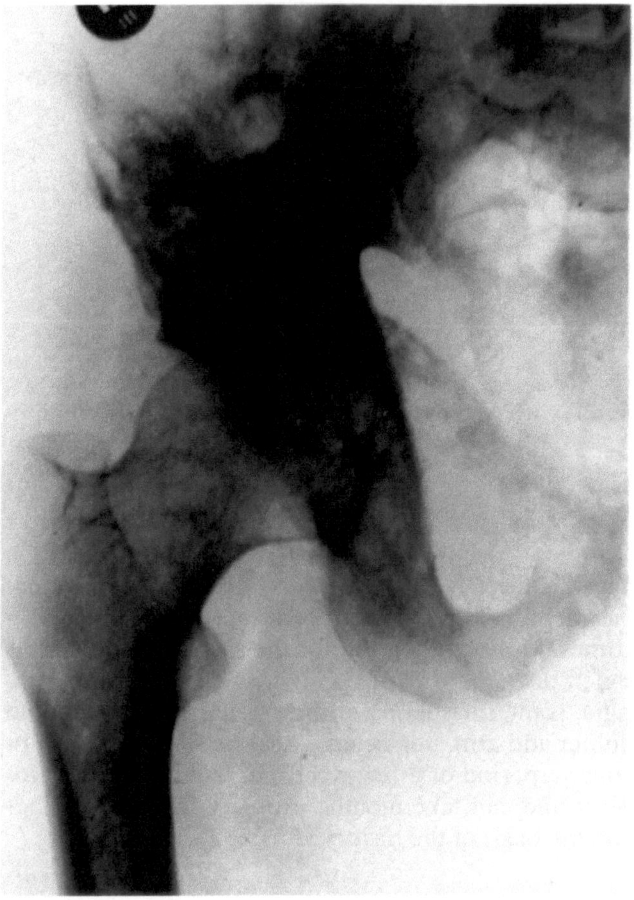

Fig. 15. X-ray of pelvis from 65 yrs. old patient with metastatic destruction of pubic bone and relevant pains. Nodular goiter. Histology of removed thyroid: follicular Ca. Later successful ^{131}I-therapy of pelvic metastasis

lesions in the skeleton or multiple metastases in the lungs, sometimes a mediastinal mass (Riccabona 1972) (Fig. 15). In such cases it is essential that with a history of thyroid surgery in the past and/or of irradiation to neck or upper chest during childhood no iodine containing contrast media should be applied during further diagnostic studies (Bauhofer 1978). In the presence of a nodular goiter thyroid malignancy should also be ruled out before other primary tumors are considered. As discussed later on, such a diagnostic approach is simple and quick, while other efforts to localize the primary lesion will be time-consuming and sometimes combined with an iodine load (constrast media!) which would finally jeopardize therapeutic possibilities for months (Bansi 1961). Considering the data presented in the first chapter one would also like to suggest, that patients with a family history of thyroid cancer – including MEN-syndromes – should be considered as likely to have thyroid cancer as long as the contrary has not been proven (Pohl et al. 1977).

Type 4:

Patients with hyperthyroid symptoms (Olen, Klinck 1965) and nodular goiter – sometimes small – are submitted to thyroid surgery after antithyroid drug preparation (Thompsen, Vinik 1983). Histology however sometimes reveals small thyroid cancer foci, occasionally in the contralateral lobe of a "toxic adenoma" or as a Graham type sclerosing microcarcinoma in a thyroid gland which – otherwise – shows all the features of classical Graves' Disease.

This effort to classify symptoms of thyroid cancer is obviously inadequate. It should rather be accepted as a vague guideline concerning the pecularities of thyroid malignancy when we have to deal with an individual patient and when we take the case history. Of course there is frequently an overlapping between types 1 and 4 or 2 and 4 and when a hypertensive patient with diarrhea, weight loss and a nodular goiter is referred to you because of "hyperthyroidism" you should think also about the possibility of medullary thyroid cancer in the context of an MEN-syndrome (Sipple 1961).

Case M.L., 59.31.05.40, female

Brother living elsewhere suffering from diarrhea and goiter, parents dead for unknown reasons. Growth of thyroid nodule in the right lobe in early spring 1975. Thyroid resection on June 18th, 1975. Histology: Medullary thyroid carcinoma. Reintervention on July 7th, 1975: Near total thyroidectomy, telecurietherapy with 60 Gy to neck. Microhemoptoe since fall 1976, chest films, endoscopy, palpation normal. 1978: calcitonin 1710 pg/ml. Liver scan, chest films, CT-scans and clinical findings normal, except BSR (33/60), no complaints. March 1980: Calcitonin 4400 pg/ml, BSR 21/46, no metastases detectable. March 1981: Coughing, chest pain. On chest film multiple metastases in both lungs. Chemotherapy with Doxorubicine – Cyclophosphamide – Vincristin for 6 cycles. December 1981 lung lesions unchanged, patient doing well. December 1981: Lymph node on the right neck side. Modified neck-dissection on January 3rd, 1983 (metastases of medullary thyroid Ca.). September 1984: Again mass in the neck, lung lesions constant, calcitonin 9000 pg/ml. Removal of local recurrence and lymph-node, telecurietherapy (20 Gy). February 1985: Increasing dyspneoa, no evidence of local recurrence, trachea free, progression of lung metastases. Ultrasound of liver regular, calcitonin unchanged. Next course of chemotherapy started. October 1985: Impaired vision left eye, dyspnoea. On bone-scans multiple metastases in the skeleton, brain-CT regular, lung lesions constant, soft tissue metastases in right breast and on the back (removed). Diarrhea (existing for years) controlled by diphenoxylate and atropin. Children of patient normal until now, in the meantime grown up and active in family business.

Probably the most essential factor in the evaluation of case histories of thyroid cancer patients is the idea in the consulted doctor's mind that the reported symptoms could also be related to the goiter of the patient, to thyroid malignancy (Huber, Riccabona 1967). We have seen patients treated for months for "obstructive lung disease" because of respiratory problems, while nobody in an endemic goiter area took notice of the very firm and already infiltrating thyroid tumor with invasion of larynx and trachea:

Case Z.H., 99.07.02.15, male

Since January 1985 swelling of the neck, dyspnoea. Treatment (elsewhere) for chronic obstructive lung disease. In April increasing respiratory distress. Radiography reveals severe tracheal compression due to a mass in the neck and (by tomography) an endotracheal tumor growth leaving only 2–3 mm of tracheal diameter. Also compression of the cervical oesophagus, multiple lung metastases. Therefore tracheostomy on April 25th, 1985 through a large immobile tumor mass. Histology: Anaplastic thyroid carcinoma (with a few papillary structures). Telecurietherapy (60 Gy) and chemotherapy, gastrostomy. Then partial remission with significant shrinking of the neck tumor, no ^{131}I-uptake, in September 1985 signs of skull metastases, chemotherapy continued. Telecurietherapy on skull basis (17 Gy). Death in October 1985 due to local tumor progression (hemorrhage by vessel invasion).

Concerning hoarseness it should be stressed – as mentioned later on – that a spontaneous recurrent nerve paralysis in the presence of a nodular goiter and a normal chest film must be considered as a manifestation of thyroid cancer until the contrary has been proven by careful histological examination of the excised thyroid nodule on the side of the damaged recurrent laryngeal nerve (Fasching 1984).

The symptom "pain in the thyroid area" can be related to thyreoiditis as well as to thyroid cancer. It should always be an argument for a thorough diagnostic evaluation of such thyroid glands as described below. Occasionally pregnant patients are seen with the growth of a goiter during pregnancy (Riccabona 1973). Per se, such observations cannot be considered essential for the existence of thyroid cancer, as it is known that the endocrinological situation in pregnancy can – in addition to other goitrogenic influences – provoke the growth of the thyroid (Bansi 1955). If nodules exist, they should, however, also be studied carefully to rule out thyroid malignancy even as no correlation between pregnancy and thyroid cancer has been shown so far (Rosvoll, Winship 1965).

It should finally be stressed that – all over the world – *symptoms* will motivate a patient to see his doctor, who – taking a careful and comprehensive history – will play a crucial role for the further fate of thyroid cancer cases if he is aware of the possible manifestations of this disease.

2 Physical Findings

The typical findings were also described decades ago (Wilson 1921): Firm, sometimes tender nodules within the thyroid, decreased mobility of the thyroid on swallowing, even exulceration in the area of the tumor (Fig. 16), lymph nodes in the neck etc. (Table 20). Spontaneous unilateral vocal chord paralysis at indirect laryngoscopy, congestion of veins around the upper thoracic aper-

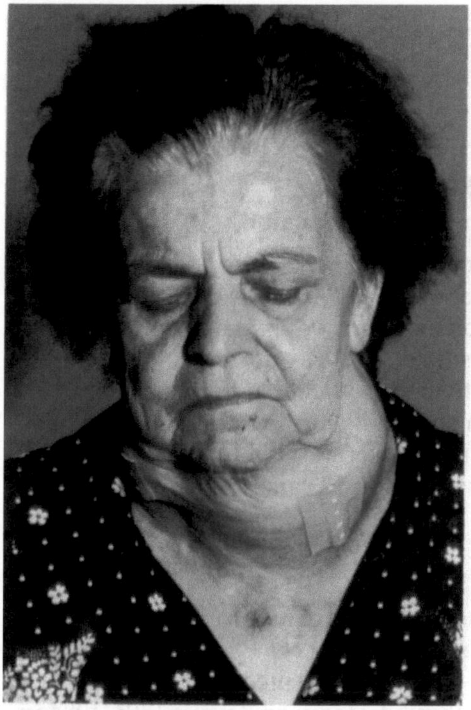

Fig. 16. Patient with rapidly growing malignant goiter, beginning exulceration on the left (covered) and near sternal notch

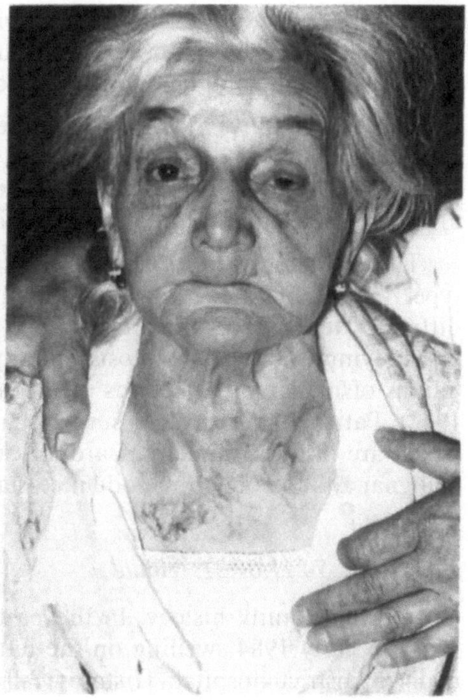

Fig. 17. Horner's syndrome on the left in patient with thyroid Ca on the left side, mediastinal mass with upper venous congestion

Table 20. Symptoms and signs of thyroid Ca.

I. Clinical Exam
  A. History
    1. Recent goiter growth
    2. Hoarseness
    3. Pain in goiter or retrauricularly
    4. Weight loss
    5. Fatigue
    6. Dyspnea
    7. Appearances of lymph nodes in the neck or submandibular area
    8. Pain in spine
    9. Ischialgia
    10. Paresis without history of vascular disease, trauma, or encephalitis
  B. Physical
    1. Thyroid nodule with increased firmness; reduced mobility; invasion of neck muscles, submandibular or cervical lymph nodes
    2. Recurrent nerve palsy on side of nodule; tenderness of thyroid nodule; Horner's syndrome on side of thyroid nodule; tenderness of one or more vertebrae; tenderness of part of the pelvis; tumor on skull

ture and Horner's syndrome may provide further evidence for thyroid malignancy (Fig. 17). The old criteria (Breitner 1960) for defining clinically a neck tumor as belonging to the thyroid should – especially in our days – be recalled:

a) The tumor moves at least to some extent when the patient swallows or coughs,
b) the carotid artery pulse can be felt behind the tumor,
c) the sternocleidomastoid muscle lies in front of the tumor.

These findings are in general easy to register in patients with histories of type 1 and 2. In type 3, however, the interpretation of physical findings can be difficult. Neck tumors in goitrous areas outside the nodular goiter can also represent lymph node tuberculosis, aneurysms of the carotid artery or manifestations of malignant affections of the reticuloendothelial system (Steiner et al. 1962). Patients after thyroid surgery can show up with extrathyroidal nodules which are in fact granulomas around suture material without any evidence of malignancy and not lymph node metastases of thyroid cancer:

Case R.M., 74.11.07.21, female

No relevant family history. In the past sometimes treated for "hyperthyroidism". In early 1984 swelling on the left side of the neck. Excision of a lymph node in district hospital: Histologically metastasis of medullary thyroid carcinoma (July 25th, 1984). Then near total thyroidectomy on August 17th, 1984 in district hospital. Histology: Medullary thyroid carcinoma (Fig. 5). Postoperatively BSR 24/51, patient feeling well, on ^{131}I-scan uptake in small thyroid remnants and in a lesion below the upper thoracic aperture on the left. Chest films and sonography regular. Telecurietherapy (60 Gy) and ^{131}I-therapy (110 mCi), calcitonin and thyroglobulin since then normal, patient doing well, no evidence of metastases or recurrence by clinical, radiological and scintigraphic exam.

The clinical picture of patients with distant metastases of thyroid cancer is even more difficult to interpret (Russell et al. 1963). The patients may have some swelling in a bone area (Fig. 18) and the tumor can pulsate as a sign of intense vascularity, so that – if e.g. localized in the sternum – one might also consider an aneurysm:

Case T.M., 90.05.11.19, female

Since 1975 pain in right chest and especially in right hip. Therefore finally exam in medical service, where osteolytic lesions were found in ribs (right) and in the ileosacral area on the right. Also destruction of vertebrae in dorsal spine, lung metastases. Biopsy of palpable tumor in the right iliac region: follicular Ca. Therefore radical thyroidectomy on March 27, 1979, where a cold nodule on the right side was removed, which proved to be the primary tumor. Postoperatively ^{131}I-therapy, telecurietherapy on iliosacral joint and neck as well as ribs, supplemented by chemotherapy (Doxorubicin, Vinblastin). With further radioiodine therapies doing well until 1982, when metastases were progressive in skeleton and lungs. Finally death with disseminated metastases in 1985.

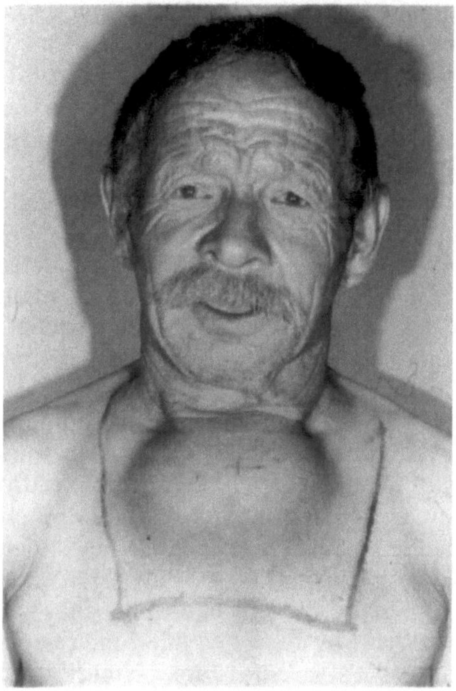

Fig. 18. Cretin with pulsating mass in upper half of sternum. Biopsy reveals follicular thyroid carcinoma

In summary a case in which a long standing goiter was not primarily related to the patients symptoms, which occurred due to bone metastases and lung metastases of follicular thyroid carcinoma. Surgery, radioiodine therapy and chemotherapy could control the disease for years but finally no definite cure could be achieved due to the already initially large tumor masses and the patient died of thyroid carcinoma.

Under these conditions it is no wonder that "biopsies" to clarify the nature of such lesions can end up as major interventions without being radical but with many units of blood required to get the patient off the operating table in decent shape! Other patients with secondary bone lesions will show only some impairment of mobility, sciatic nerve irritation or similar syndromes. Pathological fractures in the spine can – of course – produce neurological defects and even paraplegia, the rare cerebral metastases produce a pattern of clinical findings according to their localization:

Case K.R., 50.12.08.09, female

Rapid growth of goiter during pregnancy 1953. Therefore bilateral thyroid resection 1954. Histology: "Some atypical areas" in specimen. 1961: suspicion of malignant recurrent goiter. Near-total thyroidectomy on October 11th, 1961. Histology: badly differentiated follicular Ca., postoperative recurrent nerve paralysis on the left. 37 mCi ^{131}I on November 29th, 1961. January 1962: Metastases in right lower chest (lungs and below), later defined as lesion in right kidney. Right nephrectomy on March 12th,1962, 80 mCi ^{131}I on March 23 rd,

1962. Conventional radiotherapy. January 1963: Patient doing well, lung lesions constant. 123 mCi ^{131}I on March 12th, 1963, uptake in lung lesions. Again doing well, in November 1963 increased ^{131}I-retention, therefore another 100 mCi of ^{131}I on November 27th, 1963. In January 1964 dizziness, slight anisocoria (right > left), EEG regular. On scan suspicion of ^{131}I-uptake in left basal region in the skull. 120 mCi ^{131}I on April 27th, 1964. Death due to acute cerebral symptoms on the same day. Postmortem: Hemorrhage in cerebellar metastases of thyroid Ca., lung lesions fibrotic.

Lung metastases are scarcely detected by clinical exam, pleural carcinosis with effusions can be detected by auscultation and percussion.

Liver metastases are not frequent in thyroid cancer (Schauer 1984), they can, however, be detected by palpable enlargement of the liver (Fig. 19). According to some reports they can occur at a rate above normal in medullary thyroid carcinoma. It is therefore important to know, in which regions or organs thyroid cancer develops metastases most frequently (Table 21). In cases with a suspicion of some type of MEN-syndrome (see above), inspection of the buccal mucosa, blood pressure values and clinical signs of hyperparathyroidism (Ellenberg et al. 1962) can also help to guide the consulted doctor to a correct diagnosis.

Finally I would like to say that with all the diagnostic potential of modern medicine as described later, the responsibility to suspect thyroid malignancy in any of it's varieties rests primarily on the physician first consulted by the pa-

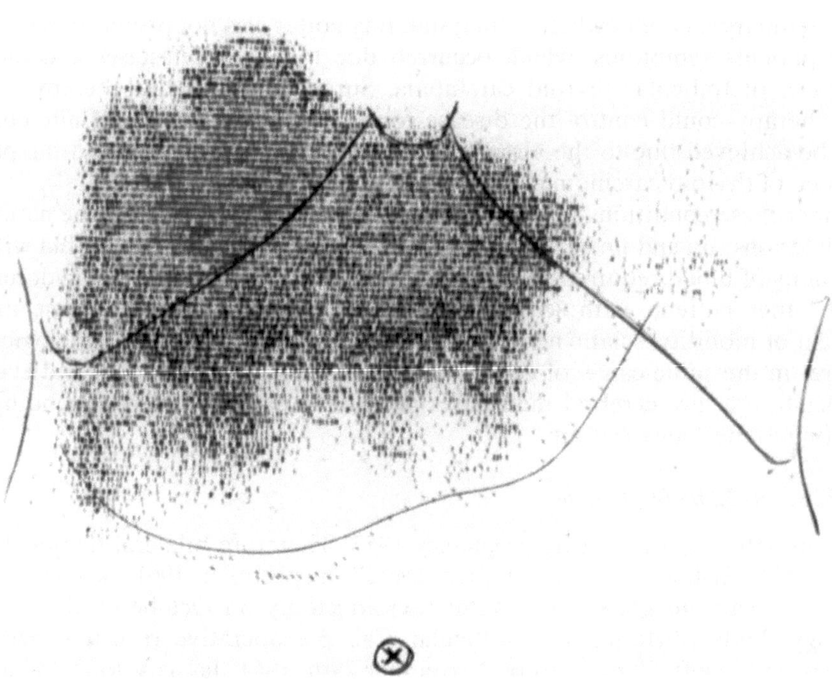

Fig. 19. Liver scan of patient with follicular thyroid Ca and liver metastases. Liver enlarged, nodular, cold areas on scan

Table 21. Sites for metastases of thyroid cancer

	Lymph-nodes	Lungs	Bone	Liver	Brain	Other
Papillary Ca.	+++	+	+	+	?	+
Follicular Ca.	+	+++	+++	+	?	?
Medullary Ca.	+++	++		++	?	?
Anaplastic Ca.	++	+++	+	+	?	?
Lymphoma	+	?	+	+	?	?

(+++ = > 15% of metastases, ++ = > 10% of metastases, ? = no reliable data available)

tient. The informations given on the last few pages should help any doctor, to think about thyroid cancer when – after talking with the patient – relevant findings are observed at a thorough physical examination. It is a guess – but I would suggest that it is a good one – that with appropriate knowledge 70% of thyroid cancer cases could be brought to appropriate therapy in time just on the basis of the informations given in 6.1 and 6.2.

3 Diagnostic Methods

Among a wide variety of possibilities for assessing the nature and extent of malignant thyroid disease it must be stressed that readily available diagnostic techniques employed by doctors and/or technicians with the appropriate knowledge should be chosen in the first place. There exist preliminary reports showing the impact of nuclear magnetic resonance imaging on the definition of thyroid lesions (Fig. 20) (Miyata et al. 1986) and pathologists are starting to use immunohistochemical techniques to clarify the nature of a thyroid fine needle aspiration specimens (Granier et al. 1986). Where, when and at what cost will such diagnostic possibilities be available on our planet, providing a rapid and adequate treatment for a thyroid cancer case? Oliver Cope (Cope 1962), the late,

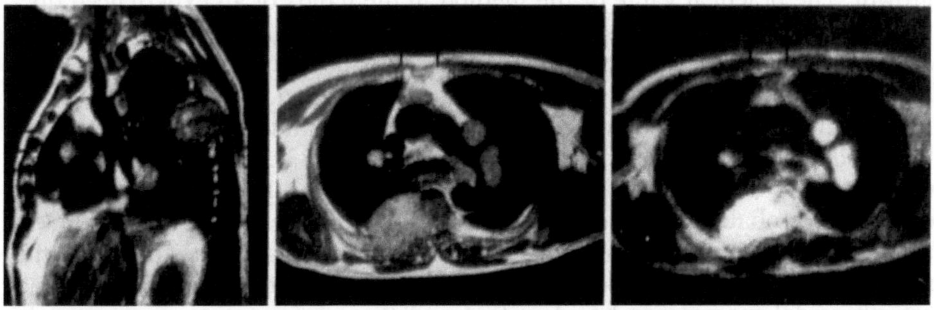

Fig. 20. NMR studies of patient with thyroid Ca and multiple metastatic lesions in lung and chest. Note clear distinction of metastatic foci in chest and lung, primary tumor with mottled spin echos (T_1)

famous endocrine surgeon once told me: "If you have proven hyperparathyroidism forget all the rest of diagnostic techniques! All the patient needs is a good surgeon!" This statement can be applied to thyroid cancer only in part because the diagnosis alone of thyroid malignancy can be difficult (see above and below). Therapeutic strategy can depend in many cases on an optimum diagnostic information before any surgical intervention. The following description of diagnostic methods in suspected thyroid cancer patients does not represent an order per se considering the value of each diagnostic method. It is rather a presentation of commonly available diagnostic procedures which – all together – can provide a definition of the existing thyroid lesion and it's extent and can therefore also promote adequate therapy.

At this point it should be mentioned, however, that diagnostic programs for "staging" of suspected thyroid malignancy can contribute significantly to reasonable therapy planning (Werner 1969), on the other hand staging is worthless in an almost suffocating patient with thyroid cancer and one should do the best to relieve – if possible – the patient of his respiratory distress without asking questions about possible metastases to bone, liver etc. So, considering all the practical limitations of diagnostic methods concerning thyroid cancer in it's different types and manifestations all over the world we should still present the most important and most accurate diagnostic techniques available today.

Ultrasound

This, non-invasive, widely available method without radiation exposure of the patient has gained wide recognition in the last 15 years for it's application in thyroid disease (Thijs 1971). Usually nodular changes in the thyroid can be identified by experienced examiners by echotomography with a 5–7 MHZ transponder with or without water filter in the neck (Fig. 21). Echostructures, however, are not typical of thyroid cancer per se: Not only have echopoor nodules been described as being consistent with thyroid malignancy (Maier 1984), but also inhomogenous echostructures within a nodular lesion and normal or echorich patterns were found to be malignant in a considerable number of cases (Frank 1980). Irregular outlines of nodular lesions are indicating of infiltrating growth. The practical value of the method in the hands of an experienced doctor lies in the fact, that it can reveal *nodular* changes in the thyroid with a diameter of only 0.5 cm, which are frequently missed by palpation or other diagnostic techniques. If such lesions can be demonstrated, an ultrasound-guided fine needle biopsy of the nodule can be performed and cytology can provide further diagnostic information (Schwarzrock et al. 1983). At present, the diagnostic accuracy of ultrasound thyroid scanning per se for the detection of thyroid cancer can probably be rated at $\sim 60\%$. The method is extremely important to assess anatomical relations of suspected malignant lesions to other organs in the neck non-invasively (Maier 1984): Carotid arteries, jugular veins, trachea and extrathyroidal masses can be identified and these informations can not only help in the diagnosis of thyroid cancer but also in planning the therapy. Mediastinal masses are difficult to delineate with ultrasound techniques, even if

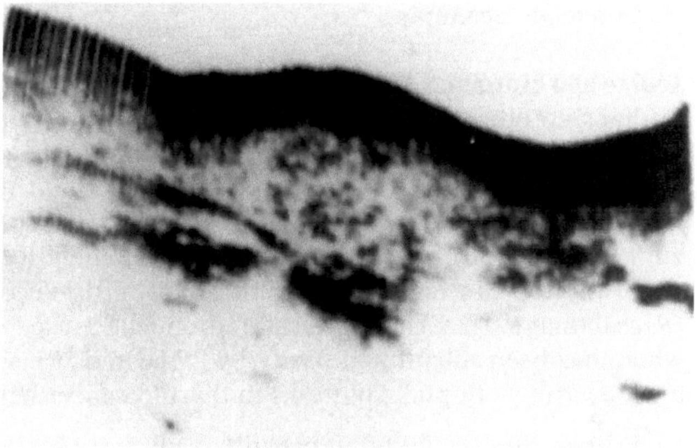

Fig. 21. Sonogram of thyroid carcinoma: nodule on right side, longitudinal section showing decreased echo density overall and mottled echo pattern as well as unclear delineation of nodule in regard to surrounding tissue

modified sound sources are applied (Taylor et al. 1974). Of course, all these statements are derived from basic knowledge of ultrasound diagnosis (Wells 1977): In general one can say, that echos reflect the water content of the examined structure (in blood, in edematous lesions, in body cavities containing fluid). Adequate technology (Kremkan 1980) can provide excellent pictures concerning the morphological distribution of this essential parameter in a tomographic style providing 3-dimensional imaging. As thyroid cancer in it's different types is only partially related to water content of the tissue, ultrasound must therefore be considered as an important but unspecific diagnostic method, which has considerable value only if used by experienced examiners. It is certainly also valuable in defining the nature of hepatomegaly in cases with thyroid cancer (metastases? Liver disease of other origin?)

Therefore its present clinical value for the diagnosis of thyroid cancer can be summarized as follows:

a) Non-invasive, delicate method without radiation exposure for detecting nodular changes in the thyroid (basically already practicable in any doctor's office),
b) Delineation of thyroidal masses in relation to big cervical vessels, sometimes capable of finding lymph node metastases,
c) Possibility of detection of metastases in liver, abdomen in general and – occasionally – soft tissues.

Disadvantages are:

a) Highly dependable on personal factors such as examiners technique and experience,
b) Unspecificity of echo patterns in thyroid nodules concerning the nature of the lesion,
c) Problems in delineating intrathoracic spread of thyroid cancer.

Radionuclide Scanning

Iodine and Hormone Metabolism as Basis for Scanning

Perhaps no other diagnostic report since the introduction of X-rays into medicine has left such an impact on oncology than the description of radioiodine uptake in metastases of thyroid cancer 40 years ago (Seidlin et al. 1948). Since then isotope scanning with rectilinear devices or with gamma-cameras (Feine, zum Winkel 1980) has remained a central element for the diagnosis and follow-up of thyroid cancer providing important information for therapeutic strategy (Riccabona 1977). The classical radionuclide used for the purpose was ^{131}I, which has been substituted partly by ^{99m}Tc and ^{123}I. With increasing experience a wide variety of uptake patterns in thyroid cancer have been described:

a) Primary lesion without or with reduced uptake ("cold"), no uptake in metastases (frequency ~ 87%) (Fig. 22).
b) Primary lesion "cold", metastases with increased uptake ("hot") (frequency ~5–10%) (Fig. 23). This phenomenon is mostly observed because of highly concentrating normal thyroid tissue in the surroundings of the primary lesion but no adequate tracer uptake around the metastases in liver, lungs, bone etc. As scanning somehow remains a relative description of activity distribution even secondaries with relatively low tracer uptake show up as "hot", while the primary lesion is cold compared with the surrounding normal thyroid tissue.
c) Primary lesion "hot" ("toxic carcinoma"), no uptake in metastases (Müller, Hamburger 1965). This phenomenon is seen in 1–2% of thyroid cancer cases (Fig. 24).
d) Primary lesion "warm" nodule, no uptake in metastasis, a finding which can be observed in up to 10% of thyroid cancer cases (Hamburger, Müller 1981). Such nodules show the same tracer uptake as the healthy surrounding thyroid tissue.
e) After surgical or radioiodine elimination of the thyroid uptake is found in previously cold metastases (Horst 1961) ~ 70% (Fig. 25).

Of course all these diagnostic patterns with the exception of a) are found only in thyroid carcinomas of real thyroid epithelium which have preserved the ability of the original thyroid cells to concentrate iodine or anions of a similar volume. As lesion-to-background activity ratios are crucial for the detection of metastases, iodine isotopes – which are at least partly incorporated in tyrosines and thyroglobuline in such tumors – will permit a better discrimination of malignant tissue on scans registered 24–48 hrs after application of the tracer than $^{99m}TcO_4$ with which scans have to be made ½–2 hrs after the radionuclide application. The low gamma-energy of ^{99m}Tc (140 keV) can also obliterate any information on small lesions lying deep within the body (Wagner 1974). Today ^{99m}Tc-thyroid scans are usually obtained to determine whether a thyroid nodule is cold or hot (average administered dose 1–2 mCi $^{99m}TcO_4$ = 37–74 MBq). If the nodule is cold, fine-needle biopsy of the areas can be added to provide further cytological evaluation (Galvan 1970) (see later). In general a "cold" nodule is considered by many authors in goiter-free countries to be indicative

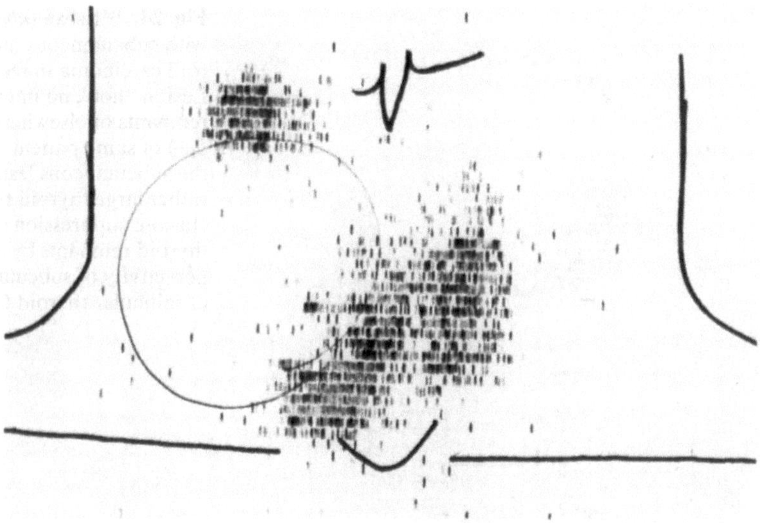

Fig. 22. ^{99m}Tc-thyroid scan showing cold area in a nodule of recent growth. Fine needle biopsy: Pap. IV. Histology: papillary Ca

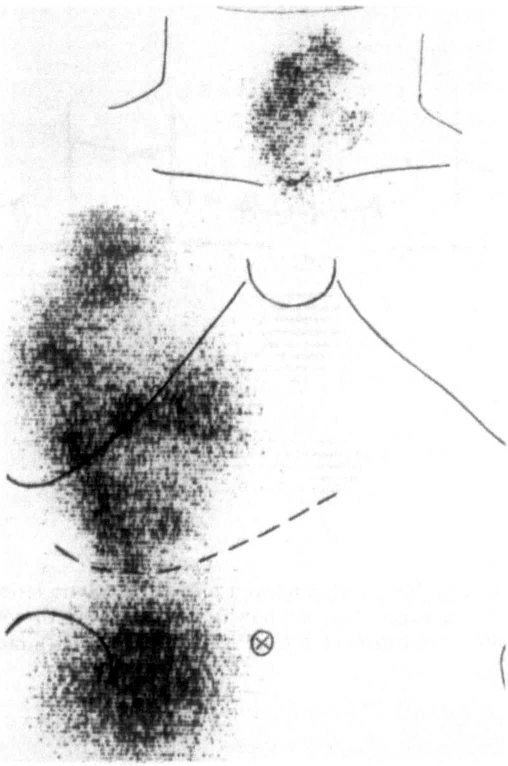

Fig. 23. Same patient as in Fig. 19: ^{131}I-scan shows "hot" spots in liver metastases and metastasis in right ilio-sacral joint. Multinodular goiter with primary lesion "cold" in relation to surrounding normal thyroid tissue. Overall primary ^{131}I-uptake in secondaries of follicular thyroid Ca

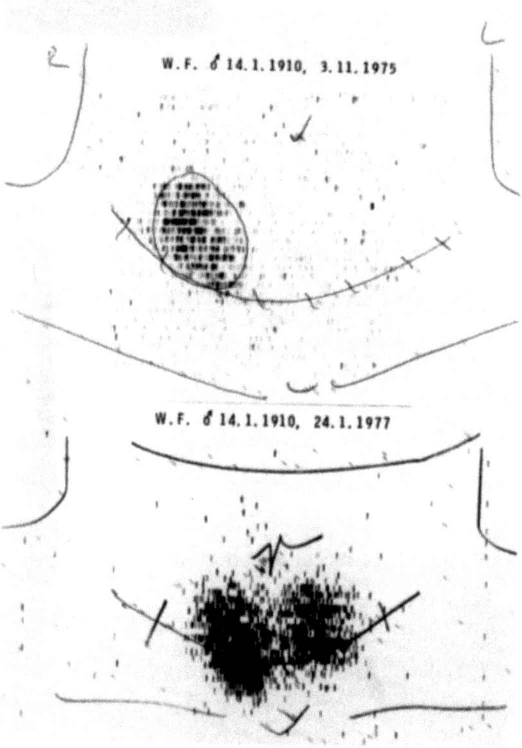

Fig. 24. ^{131}I-scan (*above*) of patient with subcutaneous metastasis of thyroid carcinoma in recurrent goiter. Lesion "hot", no uptake in thyroid remnants or elsewhere. ^{131}I-scan (*below*) of same patient after removal of the subcutaneous lesion, showing rather large thyroid remnants. Conclusion: suppression of ^{131}I-uptake in thyroid remnants by autonomous hyperactivity of subcutaneous metastasis of follicular thyroid Ca

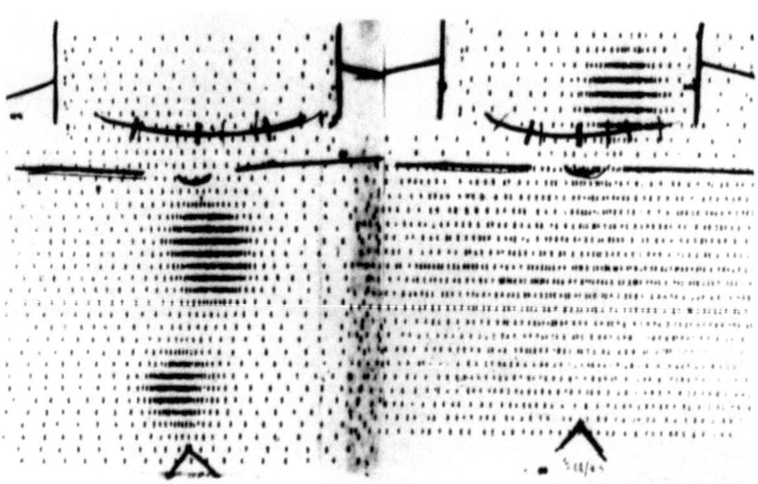

Fig. 25. *Right:* radiologically proven osteolytic lesions in sternum after thyroidectomy many years ago (histology unknown). Uptake in left thyroid remnant. No activity in sternal lesions. After elimination of thyroid remnant by ^{131}I (*left*) intense uptake of ^{131}I in sternal metastases

of thyroid malignancy so long as the contrary is not proven (Riccabona 1982). Data on the correlation of cold lesions with thyroid cancer, however, vary widely (see Table 5). As mentioned previously in the epidemiological section the incidence of thyroid cancer in cold nodules can be as high as 18% in some goiter-free countries and as low as 3% in endemic goiter countries. The "cold" nodule therefore on radioiodine or ^{99m}Tc-scans does not prove thyroid malignancy but it cannot rule it out. It should also be mentioned that ^{99m}Tc-scans register the trapping of anions in the thyroid – partly also depending on local thyroid perfusion – and can therefore be different from radioiodine scans obtained at a time in which the tracer is organically bound by true thyroid metabolism (Valenta 1966). Cases were found in which "hot" nodules on the pertechnetate-scan were cold on later radioiodine scans and were finally shown to be malignant and vice versa (Meighan, Dworkin 1969). These observations have promoted several investigators, to recommend sequential radioiodine scanning for all "hot" nodules on ^{99m}Tc-scans (Rösler 1984). We feel, however, that even this radionuclide technique will not effictively prove or rule out thyroid malignancy.

Considerable controversy exists concerning the method of radioiodine scanning in cases with suspected or proven thyroid cancer. Some groups will restrict radioiodine scanning only to patients with well differentiated thyroid carcinoma (Snyder et al. 1983), while others apply it in all cases of thyroid cancer (Riccabona 1984). This is even done in "medullary" cancer types (see previously).

Several centers and we ourselves apply diagnostic doses of 1 – 2 mCi ^{131}I (37 – 74 MBq), others insist on almost therapeutic doses of 5 – 10 and more millicuries (Hundeshagen 1983). Finally there are some groups, who do not rely on scanning, but prefer to measure whole-body retention with appropriate instruments (> 3% retention after 72 hrs in "athyroid" patients = proof of metastases with iodine uptake after application of doses of only 10 – 20 μCi of ^{131}I) (Weissel et al. 1984). It must be mentioned again, that iodine administration – be it as a contrast medium, amiodarone, broncholytic preparations, gastrointestinal tract desinfectants etc. – can block any diagnostic information from scanning in thyroid cancer patients for weeks and months (Horst 1961). The same is true of thyroid hormone preparations, with which, however, diagnostic scans are only blocked for weeks (depending on the nature of the prescribed drug) (Spencer 1978). On scanning techniques a large number of reports exists (Feine, zum Winkel 1980), discussing optimum detector systems, appropriate collimation, whole-body-profile-counting, data handling with background-subtraction etc. These are problems of nuclear medicine facilities, but any doctor treating thyroid cancer patients should know that variations in technique can also influence scan-reports and they should be especially careful to ask for scans only in patients without previous high iodine intake. In countries with extremely high nutritional iodine intake it was even suggested to put the patients on a special low- iodine diet 1 month before the scan (Barakat, Ingbar 1965). If handled and interpreted appropriately scanning with it's possible therapeutic consequences remains a basic diagnostic tool for the diagnosis and follow-up of thyroid cancer. It must also be mentioned here, that tumor tissue which concentrates radioiodine today can lose this capacity in the future and vice-versa (Riccabona et al. 1966). We therefore reject the hypothesis of some groups, that metastases of thyroid cancer with radioiodine uptake proven once, should be treated again and again with large doses of the radionuclide for years without prior diagnostic scans. Nor do we consider patients without primary radioiodine uptake in the tumor definitely "out" for further scanning and radioiodine therapy for the rest of their lives:

Case J.L., 42.11.06.65, female

Since 1982 growth of goiter, exam (elsewhere) reveals suspicion of thyroid malignancy. Near total thyroidectomy (unradical) and removal of lymph-node metastases on July 26th, 1985 (elsewhere), chest films regular. On admission (August 16th, 1985) multiple firm and quite large lymph-nodes on both sides of the neck. Scan shows ^{131}I-uptake in cervical lymph-nodes, no other ^{131}I-containing foci detectable. Modified bilateral neck dissection on August 19th, 1985. Teleradiotherapy (40 Gy) started, 120 mCi ^{131}I on August 23rd, 1985. Scans after therapy reveal not only residual lymph-node foci in the neck, but also diffuse uptake in both lungs (miliary metastases). Therefore another 150 mCi ^{131}I on September 20th, 1985.

It was also suggested that one could enhance radioiodine uptake before diagnostic scans and therapy either by administration of bovine TSH (up to 4×10 IU i.m. 8–48 hrs before application of the dose) (Horst 1985) or by prescription of thyrostatic drugs stimulating endogenous TSH-secretion for weeks (Rall et al. 1981). On the other hand we know that withdrawal of thyroid hormone after radical thyroid surgery and/or ^{131}I-therapy for an adequate period (3–6 weeks depending on the nature of the prescribed preparation: 3 weeks for triiodothyronine, 4–6 weeks for thyroxine (Tubiana 1982)) raises endogenous TSH-production to a peak and no further stimulation is necessary. Considering the possible side effects of exogenous stimulation of TSH on tracer uptake in the tumor (Thomas 1958) we never use Methimazole etc. as stimulants and only in rare cases – in which we have to save time because of clinical symptoms – do we use bovine TSH i.m. Of course one should be sure, that the patient is not pregnant when large dose scans are planned. Even as only few cases have been reported in the literature, one knows that a dose of several millicuries (= 50–100 MBq) of ^{131}I administered to a pregnant woman can produce persistent and severe damage to the thyroid of the fetus (Pfannenstiel et al. 1965). In the primary diagnosis of a thyroid nodule during pregnancy we would therefore recommend ultrasound together with fine needle biopsy and *no* isotope scan even though the usually administered doses of ^{99m}Tc must be considered as harmless for the fetus (McAfee et al. 1964). In the interpretation of scans one should be aware of a variety of possible artefacts – due to contamination of garments etc. – and possibly check the scan after decontamination, bladder voiding etc. doing either planar scintigrams in several projections with ^{131}I or SPECT with ^{123}I. It was also suggested that radioiodine retention in metastases could be estimated by adding thyroid (= neck) uptake to 48 hr urine activity (normally 93 ± 3%) of the administered dose (Horst 1961). This approach is cer-

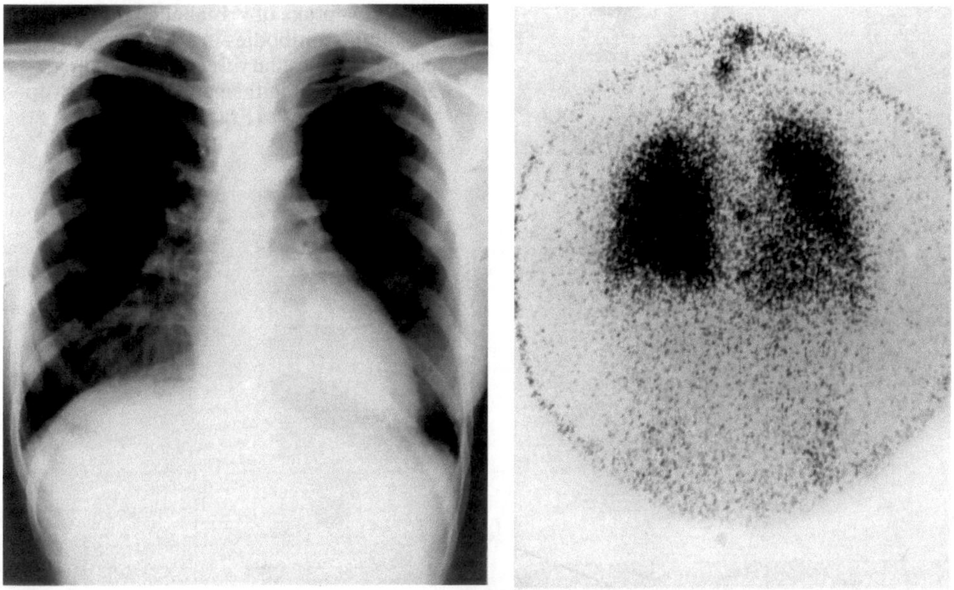

Fig. 26. Normal chest film (*left*) in patient after surgery for papillary thyroid Ca. At the same time diffuse ^{131}I-uptake in miliar lung metastases (*right*)

tainly justified on metabolic grounds, but it is prone to produce erroneous results due to incomplete urine collections. In general, isotope scanning with radioiodine is certainly no adequate substitute for an appropriate clinical follow-up, it can, however, demonstrate metastatic lesions in a well feeling patient with normal x-ray findings (Fig. 26) and point the way to adequate therapy. It can be complemented by whole body activity profile registration (Horst 1961). Another approach with radionuclide scanning on the basis of hormone metabolism in thyroid tumors seems very promising but at present – it is still in an experimental stage. It is based on the previously mentioned ability of several thyroid carcinomas to synthesize thyroglobulin without active iodide metabolism. Labelled antibodies against human thyroglobulin exist and have been used in studies showing intense uptake of this complex tracer in thyroid cancer tissue without iodide concentration (Fairwether et al. 1983) (Fig. 27). Considering the data on thyroglobulin secretion by many thyroid malignancies without radioiodine uptake (see later) this approach seems very important indeed for detection and – possibly – also for treatment of thyroid carcinoma.

Other Scanning Methods for Thyroid Cancer

For many years attempts have been made to obtain scintigraphic evidence of thyroid malignancy not only with radionuclides with an affinity to thyroid hormone metabolism but also with radiotracers with a capacity to concentrate in cancer tissue due to other biochemical properties (Horst 1985). In the 50's ^{32}P was proposed by several investigators (Ackermann, Marvin 1961), but was abandoned due to problems with the detection of it's β-rays from the outside. In

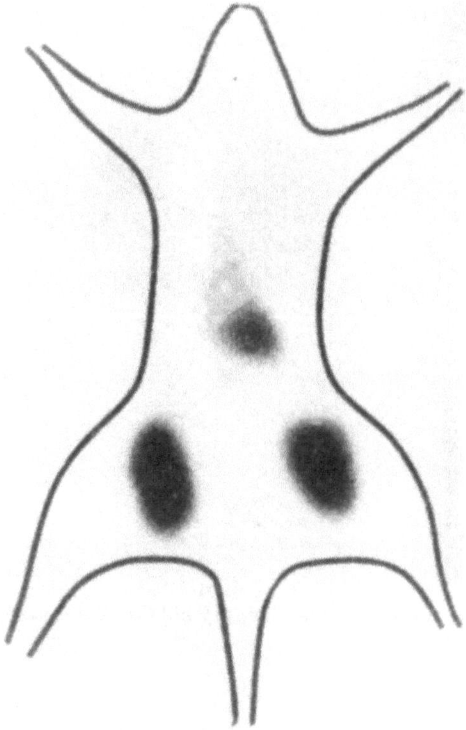

Fig. 27. Uptake of ^{131}I-labelled thyroglobulin-antibodies in rat bearing an experimental papillary thyroid carcinoma and metastases in the pelvic region. ^{131}I-uptake was negative (Fragu et al. 1983)

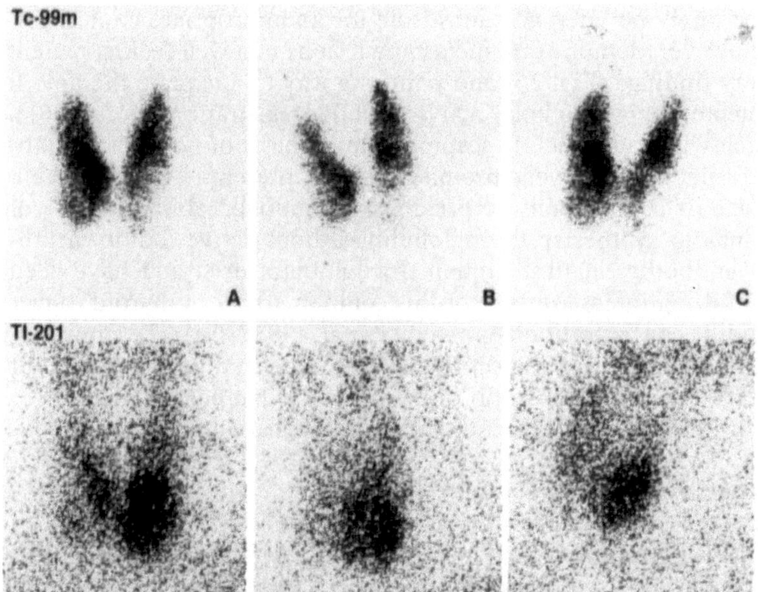

Fig. 28. ^{201}Tl-scans (*below*) and ^{99m}Tc-scans (*above*) of differentiated thyroid Ca, showing "cold" lesion in lower pole with ^{99m}Tc which is "hot" after ^{201}Tl

the late 60's ^{67}Ga-citrate was shown to accumulate in malignant thyroid tissues (scans performed 48 – 72 hrs after application of 5 mCi) (see Fig. 12) (Winchell et al. 1970). It was reported, however, that well differentiated thyroid carcinomas did not always show up as "hot" nodules on these scans and therefore in view of a diagostic accuracy of only ~ 70% and no negligible radiation exposure the method is practiced only in a few centers now. ^{201}Tl has gained interest for the scintigraphic detection of thyroid cancer in recent years (Salvatore, Mansi 1981) (Fig. 28). At present, however, the definite clinical impact of this method cannot be judged adequately: Considering the fact that ^{201}Tl acts in some way as a potassium analogue in tissue metabolism, false positive scans can be obtained in toxic adenomas, parathyroid adenomas etc. Taking into account the other diagnostic methods described previously and later on, it still remains an open question, whether ^{201}Tl scintigraphy should be included in any routine programs to assess the malignant nature of a thyroid nodule. In the last year, however, very interesting observations have been made concerning the detection of medullary thyroid carcinoma with radioiodine labelled methylbenzylguanidine (MBG) (Guilloteau et al. 1985). The tracer – usually applied for the diagnosis of phaeochromocytomas and neuroblastomas (Wieland et al. 1980) – acts as a competitor at the sites of biologically active amines synthesis. It can obviously have an affinity to medullary thyroid carcinoma cells which do not only produce the polypeptide hormone calcitonin but also serotonin etc. It is obvious, that in view of the small available patient numbers with this disease and the short and scarce experience with the radioiodine MIBG-scanning method for detection of medullary thyroid carcinoma, all relevant publications must be considered at present as "preliminary reports". The same attitude seems to apply to the use of ^{99m}Tc-DMSA (Dimercaptosuccinate) (Cole et al. 1984) and ^{131}I-CEA-antibodies (Berche et al. 1982) (Fig. 29). These diagnostic methods, however, merit continued interest in the future until definite statements on the value of the techniques can be made.

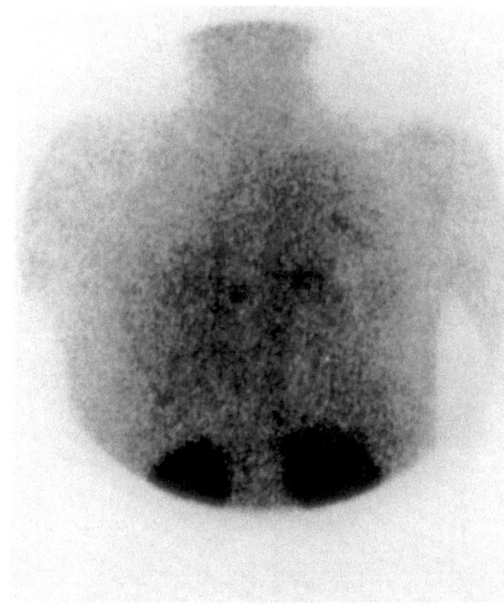

Fig. 29. Scan of chest with modified (alkaline) ^{99m}Tc-DMSA in patient with disseminated lung metastases after medullary thyroid carcinoma, showing diffuse and abnormal uptake in both lungs

Scanning of other Organs for Staging of Thyroid Cancer

Regarding the pattern of metastatic spread of thyroid cancer there are 3 methods using radionuclides for the detection of secondary lesions which can be useful today:

a) Bone Scanning

Since the introduction of ^{99m}Tc-phosphate-complexes bone scanning has become an extremely important tool for the staging of malignant tumors (Feine, zum Winkel 1980). The sensitivity of the method for the detection of bone metastases is superior to conventional radiographs, and cost and radiation exposure are lower than for a skeleton status with x-rays. As radioiodine uptake can be absent in thyroid cancer and the iodine uptake in these lesions may also change in the course of time, we recommend bone scanning after 15 mCi of ^{99m}Tc-MDP, EHDP or ^{99m}Tc-DPD (Subramanian et al. 1975) in all thyroid cancer patients with complaints like "rheumatic pain" and other skeleton-related problems. The study can be done without a period of several weeks off thyroid hormone replacement, immediately when the first such symptoms occur, and due to the physical properties of ^{99m}Tc it can also be repeated in intervals of a few months if necessary (Fig. 30). If suspicious lesions are detected by bone scanning, radiographs of the suspect areas can give more detailed morphological information (see later), and both diagnostic approaches can finally lead to an appropriate therapeutic strategy as described below.

b) Liver Scanning

In the era of sophisticated ultrasound and CT-techniques this (previously widely used) technique for the detection of liver metastases of a variety of malignant tumors has almost been forgotten in some places (Feine et al. 1979). It should be pointed out nevertheless that the combinations of ultrasound and liver scanning is about as informative as CT-scanning (Table 22), much cheaper and

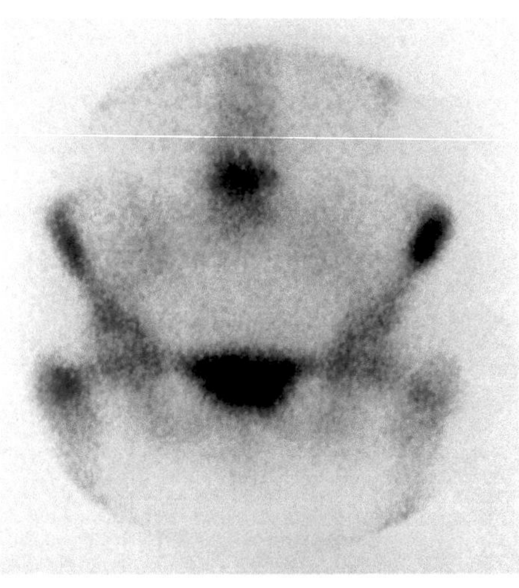

Fig. 30. Hip and spine metastases of thyroid cancer without ^{131}I-uptake but showing up as hot areas on bone scan

Table 22. Diagnostic precision of liver ultrasound, radionuclide-scan and CT (n = 110)

	Radionuclide scan	US	CT
Accuracy	79% (71–87%)	80% (72–87%)	94% (88–97%)
Sensitivity	87% (73–95%)	65% (49–78%)	89% (76–96%)
Specificity	70% (57–82%)	86% (67–94%)	95% (88–98%)

more easily available. Liver scanning in order to detect secondaries is carried out after the application of 2–3 mCi ^{99m}Tc labelled colloid in several projections using rectilinear scanners or gamma-cameras (Feine; zum Winkel 1980). Diagnostic information can sometimes be improved with single photon emission tomography (Ell 1980). As with several other cancer types, metastatic lesions in the liver impair the prognosis of relevant patients, even though these lesions can also trap radioiodine in some cases. Liver scanning should therefore be considered in thyroid cancer patients with an enlarged liver and/or with abnormal liver function parameters together with an ultrasound exam of the organ.

c) Brain Scanning

Brain metastases of thyroid cancer are rather rare (see above), they do occur, however, and therefore patients with a history of this disease and focal neurological symptoms should be studied closely to rule out secondaries as the cause of their symptoms. A proper localization of metastases, the distinction between a solitary lesion and multiple metastases are crucial parameters for therapy planning (see later). If there is no ^{131}I-uptake in the brain, this does not rule out a cerebral spread of thyroid malignancy for similar reasons as those mentioned in the section on bone scanning. If a CT-study can be done, it is certainly preferable to brain scanning due to it's superior resolution and better diagnostic accuracy. If CT-scans, however, are not available brain scintigraphy after injection of 10–15 mCi (= ~ 550 MBq) $^{99m}TcO_4$, ^{99m}Tc-Glucoheptonate and other ^{99m}Tc-labeled brain tracers (Tejero-Vidal 1979) can be used to detect metastatic lesions in the brain (Buell et al. 1978). Brain scanning performance is better when it is done with a gamma-camera as dynamic and static study (Hugl et al. 1978), than with a rectilinear scanner. CT-scans with application of contrast media should be avoided – if possible – in patients with other metastases which show ^{131}I-uptake, as the iodine exposure would prevent the treatment of the other lesions with radioiodine (see later and above).

Fluorescent Scanning (Patton et al. 1976)

The method does not require the administration of a radionuclide to the patient, it is performed with a moving, well cooled semiconductor detector which registers the fluorescence signals provoked by an ^{124}Am source moving right along with the detector over the thyroid. Appropriate collimation is essential.

The intensity of the radiation induced fluorescence phenomena depends in the thyroid on local iodine content. As it could be expected from the results of autoradiography of thyroid cancer and chemical tissue analysis, thyroid malignancies contain little iodine in general and are therefore "cold spots" on a fluorescent scan. There are, however, also many benign thyroid nodules with a reduced iodine content, which therefore show the same fluorescence distribution pattern as thyroid cancer (Hoffer et al. 1972). The only instance in which fluorescent scanning would provide additional information to ^{99m}Tc or radioiodine scintigraphy would be in cases of macrofollicular, colloid-rich nodules which are usually "hot" on fluorescence pictures and "cold" on isotope scans. The method cannot be applied for the purpose of localizing metastases in the trunk, also it's availability is rare, and therefore it never achieved the diagnostic impact of the other methods mentioned in this chapter.

Diagnosis by Thermography (Samuels 1972)
It was hoped – that as in patients with breast cancer – thermography would provide important adjunctive information to distinguish between benign and malignant thyroid nodules. Due to the normally large variations in thermographic patterns in the neck this promise, however, was not fulfilled with an adequate diagnostic accuracy (Oberdisse et al. 1980).

Diagnosis by Cytology
Considering the fact that most of the diagnostic methods so far yield only unspecific results when the patient is examined for the first time, it is not surprising that modern cytological criteria have also been applied to specimens obtained from some clinically, sonographically or scintigraphically suspect thyroid nodules (Persson 1967). As far as technique is concerned the debate between proponents of the older silverman-needle (Hamlin, Vickery 1956) approach and the newer fine needle biopsy (Galvan et al. 1984) continued for years, while some authors proposed drill biopsies (Oberdisse et al. 1980). According to our opinion this debate is irrelevant. To obtain optimum results by cytological methods you have to consider the compliance of your patients, the accuracy of the doctor obtaining the specimen while handling the technique of his choice with perfection and an experienced cytologist (which can sometimes be the same person who punctures the thyroid) who knows all the pitfalls of thyroid cytomorphology. In view of it's simplicity, it's lack of complications and it's adequate diagnostic results we have abandoned large-needle biopsy and are using the fine needle technique since 1969. Our own experience with this method is based on 15152 biopsies from 1970–1984. The technique is easy: After skin desinfection a no. 12–no. 18 gauge needle on a 10–20 ml syringe is inserted in the nodule in a plane parallel to the tracheal wall, while the examiner holds the nodule with the other hand (Fig. 31) and moderate suction is applied. The needle is then drawn back by about 1 cm and plunged again in the nodule in a different direction. This manoeuvre is repeated a few times under continuous suction. When cyst fluid is aspirated the syringe is allowed to fill and if the nodule has not disappeared after that other syringes can be adapted and filled also. If no fluid is obtained the content of the needle is put on a slide, and a smear is

Fig. 31. Fine needle biopsy of thyroid nodule no. 12 needle applied to 20 ml syringe, puncture palpable nodule, in this case aspiration of cyst fluid

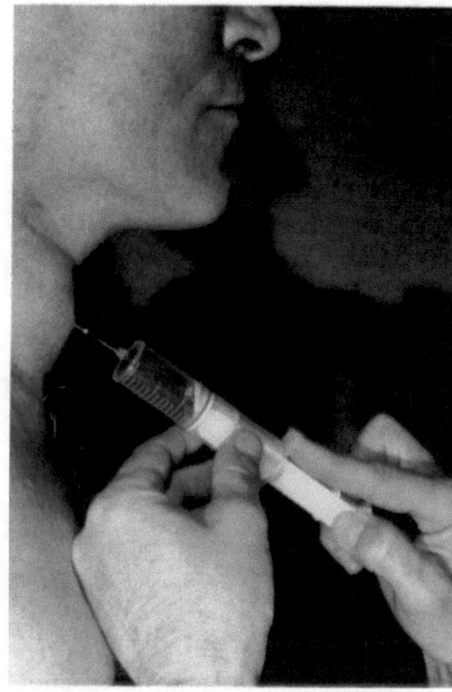

made and stained according to May-Grünwald (Droese 1979). If fluid in larger amounts is aspirated, it is centrifuged in a normal laboratory centrifuge and the pellet is used for the smear and staining. Sonography can sometimes guide the needle better into nodules than palpation. In this way it is possible to obtain specimens of several nodules in the thyroid, which can be important in multinodular goiter. As seen from Fig. 32 microscopic pictures can range from clear-cut anaplastic tumor cells to Huerthle cells with unclear dignity and hyperplasia with some nuclear irregularities which can represent either well-differentiated carcinoma or a benign hyperplastic adenoma. The problem of classification therefore always exists. While there are of course specimens from which the diagnosis of "subacute thyroiditis", "papillary carcinoma", "anaplastic carcinoma" etc. can be made, a responsible evaluation of the cell pattern in many cases will only permit a classification in "malignant", "suspect", "no evidence of malignancy" or a classification according to Papanicolaou. The practical impact of such classification systems depends mostly on the definition of "suspect" (corresponding to Pap. III or IV): We agree with those authors (Hofstädter 1983) who tend to make such diagnoses even when there are only a few criteria, which make the cells "suspect" and which involves a rather high rate of false positive cytological diagnoses, but which restricts the dangerous false negative results to a very low figure (Walfish et al. 1977). In suspect (= Pap. III, IV) cases, surgery will usually be done, or at least a close follow-up will be started and usually – in the case of cancer – appropriate therapy is anyway still done at an adequate time. If you accept, however, irregularities in thy-

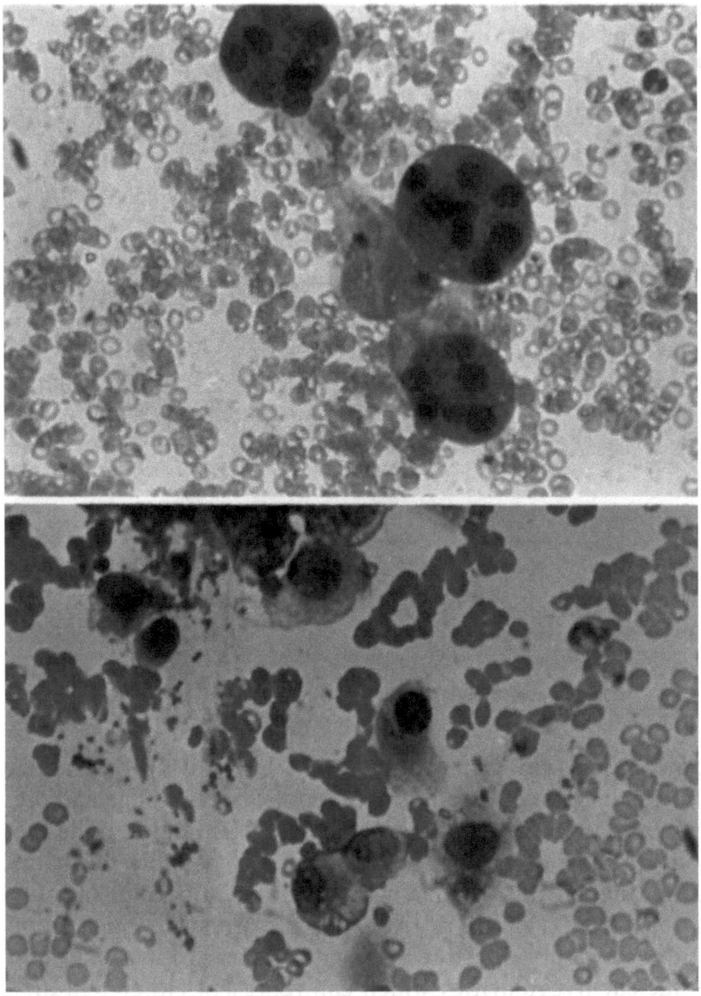

Fig. 32. Examples of cytological smears of thyroid fine needle biopsy. *Above:* subacute thyroiditis with typical giant cells. *Below:* grotesque cell configuration in anaplastic thyroid Ca

roid cell structure to a large extent simply as functionally determined criteria and hand out "benign" (Pap. II) diagnoses in such cases you are probably missing several differentiated thyroid carcinomas and those patients will eventually show up later in a prognostically worse TNM-stage for therapy:

Case R. W., 76.07.01.39, female

Removal of toxic adenoma in the right thyroid lobe on May 6th, 1981, left lobe classified as normal. Prophylaxis against goiter recurrence with 75 mcg T_4/day. In January 1985 patient notes growth of recurrent goiter on the left. T_4-dose increased to 150 mcg/day. Nevertheless further goiter growth, in June clearly extrathyroidal neck tumor. Sonography with inhomogenous echostructures, chest

Table 23. Results of fine needle biopsy

Source	n total	n histology	According to histology		
			Correct	False positive	False negative
Boey et al.	684	117	93.2%	/	6.8%
Droese	12000	440	93.7%	0.3%	6.0%
Galvan	13561	2744	75.0%	24.6%	0.4%
Own material (evaluated)	7587	991	92.0%	6.7%	0.5%

film regular. Lobectomy on the left with modified neck-dissection on the left on June 19th, 1985. Histology: Papillary thyroid Ca. Teleradiotherapy (60 Gy), 82 mCi ^{131}I on July 26th, 1985. Now thyroglobulin normal, patient doing well, no evidence of recurrence or metastases.

Even considering all these technical and evaluation problems it must be stated, that needle biopsy has become an exceedingly valuable tool in the diagnosis of thyroid cancer (Table 23) giving an average diagnostic accuracy of ~90% if performed properly (Galvan 1983). Except for some minimal hematomas and 1 infection of a cystic nodule we have seen no complications in all our biopsies. Before closing this section 2 questions should still be answered: what should one do when no appropriate material for cytological classification can be obtained from a thyroid nodule and what about the few false negative cases even in departments with excellent results overall?

Regarding the first question it should be said, that a perfect technique of performing the biopsy without too much suction in the syringe can certainly lessen the quota of unrepresentative specimens. The incidence of such "Pap. X"-specimens decreased in our series between 1970 and 1980 from 23.1 to 15.5% as a sign of better technique with increasing experience. When, however, with an optimum technique no appropriate material can be obtained, the nodule must be considered as potentially malignant until the contrary is proven either by histology at surgery or by another needle biopsy during a short-term follow-up. The false negatives can mostly be attributed to the fact that the malignant lesion was missed by the examiner (Oberdisse et al. 1980). Small carcinomas in the contralateral lobe of an impressive large cold nodule can remain undetected and in multinodular goiter there is the possibility that after puncturing 3 or 4 nodules you just miss the really malignant one. These problems can perhaps be overcome by sonography guided punctures, which might still improve overall results. As this group is probably the largest in the false negative series only few cases remain in which an erroneous diagnosis was made by the cytologist. Here again familiarity of the examiner with the structural peculiarities of thyroid cells in general and of thyroid cancer especially together with adequate experience will help to reduce these wrong classifications.

Radiological Methods

X-ray studies of chest and neck are – of course – the oldest diagnostic methods used to assess the spread and effects of thyroid cancer on surrounding structures (Ruckensteiner 1963): Deviation and/or compression of the trachea, involvement of the oesophagus, signs of retrotracheal and/or retrovisceral tumor growth, extension of the tumor into the mediastinum, lung metastases or pleural effusion due to pleural carcinosis can all be seen on such radiographs (Fig. 33). Decreased mobility of the thyroid mass on swallowing has been described as a sign of malignancy as well as microcalcifications in papillary carcinomas (Meissner, Lahey 1948). Already decades ago it was stated that the relation of a goiter to other structures in the neck could not be defined only on the basis of a routine chest film (Sgalitzer, Stöhr 1924). Fluoroscopy (today usually

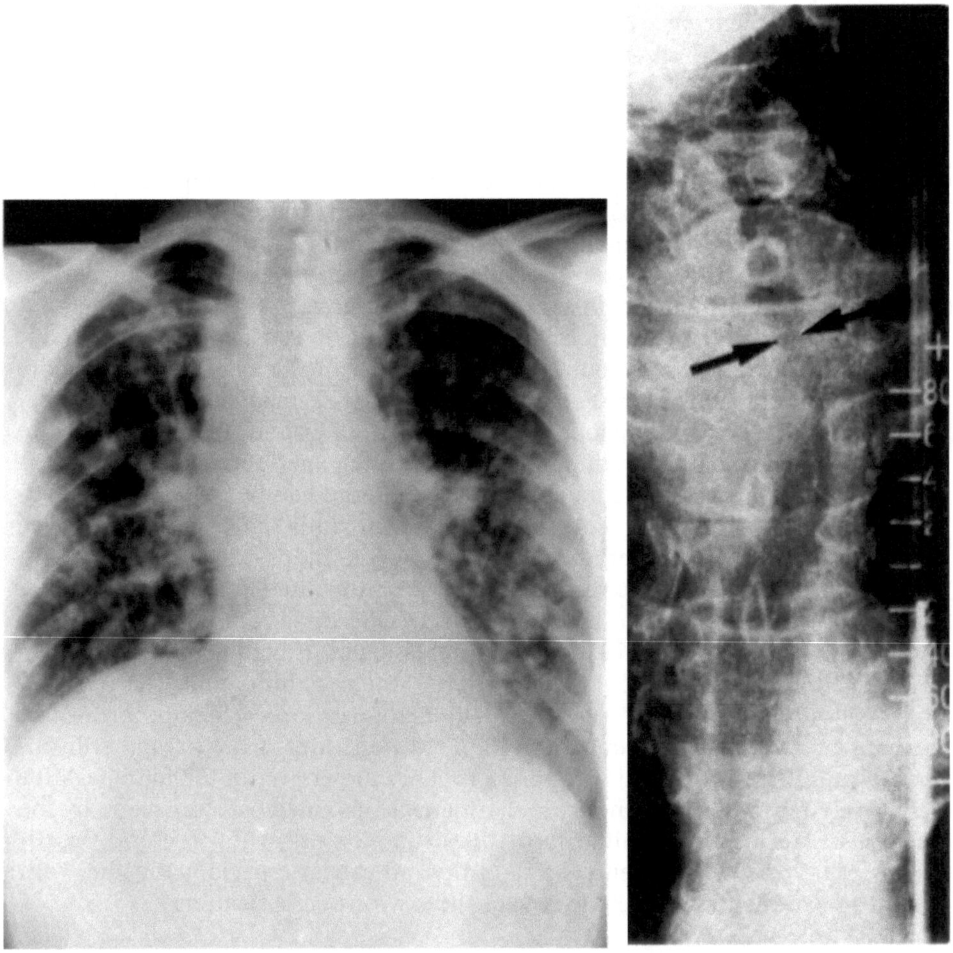

Fig. 33. Chest (*left*) and neck (*right*) films of thyroid cancer patient with tracheal stenosis and lung metastases

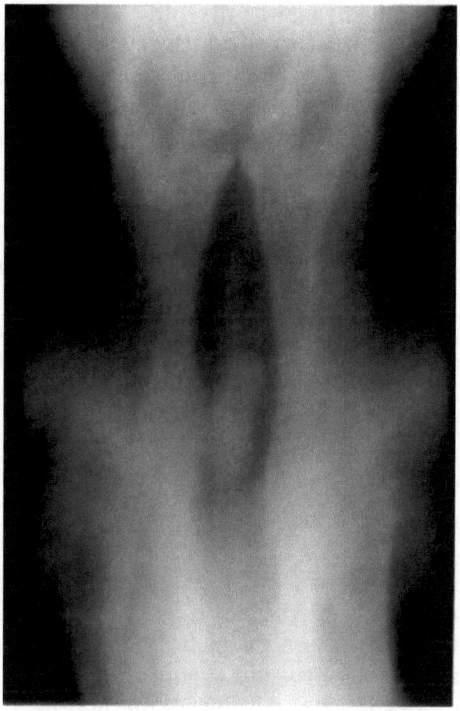

Fig. 34. Tomogram of trachea of patient with severe dyspnoea, normal trachea on regular films and endotracheal obstruction due to recurrence of thyroid Ca

with image intensifier and TV-monitor) should be done to see in which diameters the trachea is mainly affected and what the anatomy of the neck organs looks like and then representative films of the most important aspects should be made (Huber, Riccabona 1967). Endotracheal tumor growth may occasionally be seen with this technique. If the endotracheal tumor is small, however, it may be missed. Inspiratory distress with normal findings at indirect laryngoscopy and no explanation from neck and chest films taken under the guidelines mentioned above in the presence of a suspect goiter should be considered a reason for tomography of trachea and mediastinum (Fig. 34), which will then sometimes reveal intratracheal masses, leaving only a few millimeters of the tracheal diameter free for respiration:

Case A.E., 02.31.10.40, female

October 1967: Thyroid resection on the right for single nodule for cosmetic reasons (elsewhere) without evidence of malignancy in the specimen. In spite of postoperative thyroid medication growth of recurrent nodular goiter (nodules "cold"), therefore reintervention in November 1971: Obviously malignant tumor with invasion of the tracheal wall, palliative near-total thyroidectomy (postoperatively recurrent nerve paralysis on the right side). Histology: Papillary Ca. Teleradiotherapy (60 Gy), 100 mCi ^{131}I in December 1971. Then remission until summer 1974: Increasing dyspnoea, sometimes acute respiratory problems. Endoscopy and tomogram of trachea and chest: Lungs free, endotracheal recurrence of thyroid Ca. with severe narrowing of tracheal diameter. Reintervention on July 11th, 1974: Removal of local recurrence with resection of parts of the trachea, tracheal defect covered by free transplant from nasal septum. Postoperatively chemotherapy, as no ^{131}I-uptake detectable. January 1975: Recurrence at sternal notch reaching down to mediastinum, dyspnoea. Sternotomy, removal of the recurrent tumor, teleradiotherapy (40 Gy) to upper chest, 150 mCi ^{131}I. May 1977: Respiratory distress, recurrence within the trachea, also tracheal stenosis due to scar formation, tracheostomy, chemotherapy. November 1977: subglottic tumor progressive, metastases in sternum, chemotherapy continued. March 1979 further progression of endotracheal tumor growth and of sternal metastases: Teleradiotherapy (40 Gy), chemotherapy. Increasing hemoptoe and dyspnoea, weakness, death on May 22nd, 1980 due to hemorrhage from mediastinal tumor metastases with invasion of trachea and large intrathoracic vessels.

Tomography of the mediastinum and the chest can also help to delineate intrathoracic tumor masses, which is extremely important for therapeutic planning. We know that x-rays are absorbed according to the density of tissue they penetrate. Air in the trachea and in the lungs is a wonderful "contrast medium" in this regard, while an opacity will be seen in any tissue with greater density regardless of whether it is a tumor, scar, or a thick blood filled vessel and therefore the nature of such "shadows" needs further definition by the other diagnostic approaches mentioned in this chapter. On the other hand there is no more simple and accurate method for correlating dyspnoea with the mechanical effects of a benign or malignant goiter, giving at the same time important information on other possible reasons for breathing difficulties. It was shown (Fuchsig et al. 1963), that a narrowing of the tracheal diameter by more than ⅓ increases resistance to breathing significantly and can therefore be responsible for dyspnoea. Dysphagia – as sometimes reported by goiter patients – can be attributed to an effective impairment of the oesophagus by a thyroid mass only in a few instances as the oesophagus is a muscular, elastic organ capable of retaining it's function even when deviations or moderate pressure on it exist (Huber 1958). A barium swallow can easily delineate invasion of the oesophagus by a malignant thyroid tumor and – in severe cases – demonstrate oesophago-tracheal fistula. It has already been mentioned that affections of the mediastinum, lungs and pleural cavities can be seen on chest films. Dyspnoea in the presence of heart disease or severe emphysema can also be explained without impairment of the trachea. Radiology overall provides valuable information for the "staging" of thyroid cancer too. This is especially important with regard to bone metastases. Bone scans (see above) play a crucial role as a screening method for the existence of such lesions, but their exact anatomical location, and the possibility of surgical treatment are and will remain questions to be answered by the radiologist. Detailed x-ray studies (possibly including tomography) of scintigraphically suspect areas in the skeleton (Fig. 35) are essential in these cases for an appropriate diagnosis and therapy planning. Of course all the pitfalls of radiological exams of the skeletal system must be known (Shafer, Tully 1974) in order to interpret findings correctly and to avoid either unnecessary therapeutic efforts or therapeutic neglect. It should be known – e.g. – that

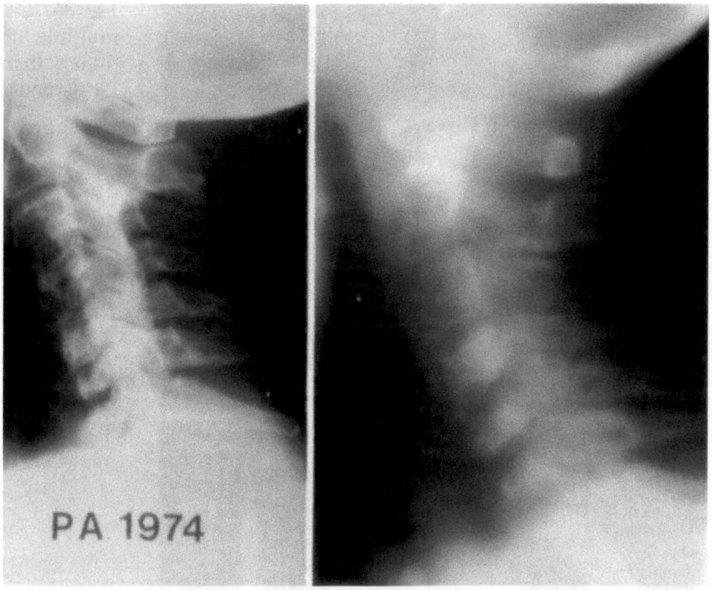

Fig. 35. Tomogram of osteolytic metastasis of thyroid Ca in cervical spine with beginning paraplegia

the diagnosis of metastases in the sternum or in the skull can be made only if clinical, scintigraphic and detailed x-ray results correlate. Another warning should be put forth once again, against the use of iodine containing contrast media. If bone or other metastases of an unknown primary tumor are detected in a patient with nodular goiter the thyroid pathology should be studied and assessed before such contrast media are applied in the search for other possible locations of the primary lesion! The reason for this argument has been mentioned previously, and it is especially valid for myelography and lymphography as the contrast media used in such studies can block radioiodine uptake in metastases of thyroid cancer not only for weeks or a few months but even for years (Börner 1976)! Depending on the amount given, contrast media used for angiography or pyelography are usually eliminated more rapidly, so that approximately 3 months after such a study radioiodine can be used for diagnosis and therapy (Schicha et al. 1980). In locations in which bone scans are not readily available a radiological skeleton status (skull, spine, pelvis) can be substituted for the scintigraphic bone exam even as cost and radiation exposure are higher (Zechmann et al. 1981).

Another very important contribution of radiology to the diagnosis of thyroid cancer is CT-scanning (Hermann et al. 1985). Even as this method – especially when used without contrast media – will only rarely be essential for the diagnosis of the primary thyroid tumor, it is extremely important to assess intrathoracic spread of the disease and to define single or multiple metastases in lungs, liver and brain (Fig. 36). As with conventional radiological methods small metastases in the lungs can be missed, as – especially in obese patients –

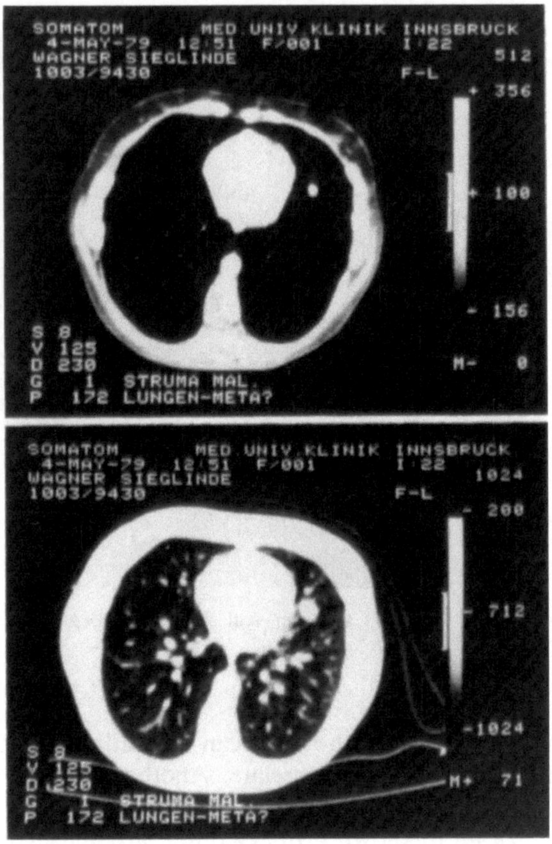

Fig. 36. CT-scans of chest showing multiple lung metastases of medullary thyroid Ca, normal chest x-ray regular

sonography of the liver is sometimes difficult to interpret and isotope scanning of brain and liver has only a limited resolution, CT-scans should – if possible – be carried out in any patient in whom the radioiodine scan is normal after primary treatment and some clinical or laboratory suspicion remains concerning the growth of metastases.

With all the merits of the diagnostic methods of radiology (including CT-scanning) and Nuclear Medicine it should be remembered, that all these studies subject the patient to some radiation exposure (Hundeshagen 1980) and therefore one should consider this problem with regard to the follow-up programs of patients with thyroid cancer: Of course all these methods should be avoided in pregnant women without vital necessity, as the applied doses might harm the fetus. Modern diagnostic systems used in radiology and nuclear medicine have permitted to reduce the radiation dose to the patient considerably (Brill 1982). As long as adequate diagnostic information can be obtained without the use of ionizing radiation one should restrict the radiological and Nuclear Medicine procedures to a clinically justified minimum, as patients with thyroid cancer will frequently remain in regular follow-up programs for a decade or more (see later).

In Vitro Diagnostic Methods

Chemical Methods

Besides routine determination of calcium concentrations in serum after surgery for thyroid cancer and occasional liver function tests (GOT, GPT, alc. Phosphatase, γGT) during follow-up studies for the possibility of liver metastases only carcino-embryogenic antigen (CEA) determined by immunochemical methods (Weissel, Höfer 1983) has gained some significance in the follow-up of medullary or anaplastic thyroid cancer (Busnardo et al. 1983). This tumor marker can also be measured in blood by radioassay as discussed later on. Thyroxine and TSH can also be quantified by enzyme immunoassays and these values can help to assess the functional status regarding thyroid hormone concentrations in blood after treatment or under substitution therapy. Also these parameters can be obtained by radioassays.

Thyroid autoantibodies as determined by agglutination tests (Boyden 1951) against thyroglobulin and/or microsomal antigens can be valuable indicators in the differential diagnosis between autoimmune thyroiditis and thyroid cancer. High autoantibody titers (> 1:320 for thyroglobulin autoantibodies = TGA, or > 1:400 for microsomal autoantibodies = MSA) are a classical feature of active Hashimoto's disease, while lower titers can occasionally also occur in thyroid cancer (DeGroot et al. 1977): One should keep in mind that – as mentioned previously – lymphosarcoma can (in rare cases) be seen together with Hashimoto's thyroiditis and therefore firm nodular goiters in the framework of autoimmune thyroiditis, which do not respond to medical therapy promptly (Lindsay, Dailey 1965) should be considered as suspicious. Another important application of such hemagglutination tests is the detection of disturbing thyroid autoantibodies for thyroglobulin radioassays in follow-up programs as evidence of relevant autoantibody titers against thyroglobulin of course inhibits the interpretation of radioimmunoassays to measure the antigen thyroglobulin (Baschieri et al. 1981).

Radioassays

Of course competitive protein binding assays to measure T_4- and T_3-uptake in serum were of value in checking the thyroid hormone dose after surgery and/or ^{131}I-treatment for thyroid cancer (Oberdisse et al. 1980). Today T_4, free T_4-indices, free T_4, T_3, free T_3 or reverse T_3 are mostly determined by radioimmunological methods (Ellis, Ekins 1973, Hall et al. 1971) for these purposes, as well as TSH before or after TRH. It is also important to know these values to check the ablative effect of ^{131}I-therapy as discussed later on. As functional abnormalities regarding the total hormone supply to the body are not typical features of thyroid cancer, these methods will scarcely be valuable for the primary diagnosis of thyroid malignancy. Therefore the technique of assays will not be discussed here in detail, relevant information can be obtained from the endocrinological literature (Klein et al. 1978) where also pitfalls in the interpretation of such assays are mentioned. Some details of test interpretation during the follow-up studies of thyroid cancer will be mentioned in the relevant chapter in this booklet. There are, however, a few radioimmunoassays, which have earned a reputation as "tumor markers" for thyroid cancer (Horst 1985). The most important ones used for the diagnosis of thyroid cancer are presented in alphabetical order, which does not reflect the frequency in which they are requested but does reflect their historical development.

a) Carcino-embryonic Antigen (CEA)
In some regards this "tumor marker" is just the opposite of the substance mentioned in the next section (calcitonin): It is a substance which is normally produced in the fetus, then it's blood concentrations drop to extremely low levels (< 0.5 ng/ml) 3 months after birth. They increase in adult life when a variety of malignancies occur (Lawrence et al. 1972): This feature even gave rise to hopes, that by a relatively simple radioimmunoassay or enzyme immunoassay the diagnosis of cancer could be established. We all know by now that these hopes have not been fullfilled, we know also on the other hand that CEA is a valuable tumor-marker for colo-rectal carcinoma, for ovarian cancer and last but not least for thyroid cancer (Ishikawa, Hamada 1976) and several other neoplasms. In thyroid cancer elevated values were reported in cases with medullary carcinoma and anaplastic carcinoma. The substance therefore lacks the specificity of calcitonin, it may, however, be present in abnormal amounts in the blood of thyroid cancer patients where other relevant "tumor markers" cannot be detected. False negatives occur in up to 30% (Calmette et al. 1978), false-positives were mainly traced to the existence of second neoplasms (e.g. in the colon) or to smoking. Today CEA-assays are usually done in combination with calcitonin or with thyroglobulin in patients with a suspicion of thyroid cancer or during follow-up programs, where they can help to monitor the course of the disease (see later).

b) Calcitonin-radioimmunoassay (Thyrocalcitonin)
After it was established that medullary thyroid carcinoma produces and secretes calcitonin (Williams 1966), several groups tried hard to develop a sensitive and specific radioimmunoassay to measure the low concentration of this polypeptide hormone in blood (Goltzman et al. 1974) and they succeeded (Wells et al. 1975). Among all the "tumor markers" presented today in the literature there are only very few which can equal calcitonin concerning it's specificity for a well-defined tumor type. This means that any patient with an elevated calcitonin level in the blood is likely to have medullary thyroid carcinoma or at least C-cell hyperplasia, which is considered by some authors as precancerosis (Wolfe, De Lellis 1981). Rarely ectopic production of calcitonin has been described. When normal values are found – e.g. in family screening programs of patients with such tumors – stimulation tests can be performed. Originally stimulation was mostly carried out by calcium infusion (15 mg of calcium/kg body weight in saline over 3 hours i.v.) (Parthemore et al. 1974), then pentagastrin stimulation (bolus i.v., 0.5 µg/kg body weight) was recommended (Wells et al. 1978) and today many groups use ethanol (Cohen et al. 1973) as a stimulant ("a glass of whisky" = 50 ml), as this method shows an adequate stimulatory effect with fewer side effects than the other techniques. Assay methods are similar for all available "kits", they are not very

simple procedures and quality control protocols (unspecific binding, inter- and intraassay variance, optimal standards) are essential for the performance of the test. On the other hand abnormal values are such sensitive diagnostic parameters, that one can be sure that a patient with elevated calcitonin more than 3 months after "radical" surgery for medullary thyroid carcinoma *must have tumor residues or metastases even if no clinical, radiological or scintigraphic evidence of persistent disease can be found:*

Case H.J., 36.14.08.11, male

Since 1978 growth of an indolent mass on the left side of the neck. No family history of goiter, no further complaints. Nodular goiter (II) with firm nodule in the left lobe. Large tumor of one cervical lymph-node on the left, nodules cold on thyroid scan, cytology equivocal, chest film regular. Near total thyroidectomy on February 2nd, 1982 with modified neck-dissection on the left. Histology: Medullary thyroid carcinoma. Teleradiotherapy (60 Gy) and 94 mCi ^{131}I on February 2nd, 1982. May 1982: Calcitonin 565 pg/ml, no other evidence of tumor recurrence or metastases. December 1982: suspect nodule in neck. Excision on January 3rd, 1983: no tumor, granuloma. May 1983: Calcitonin 729 pg/ml, patient well, no clinical evidence of tumor growth. Summer 1984: Another nodule on left neck side. Removal on July 25th, 1984: Lymph-node metastases, 111 mCi ^{131}I, March 1985: Calcitonin 3130 pg/ml. June 1985: Again nodule on left neck side, swelling of left parotid gland. Removal of neck tumor on July 3rd, 1985, parotid gland becomes normal. Chemotherapy started (Aclacinomycin). At present calcitonin levels decreasing.

In stimulation tests a rise of serum calcitonin above 90 ng/ml must be considered as suspicious of medullary thyroid carcinoma even if basal values are normal as it is known that so far no false positive results have been recorded, but that in ~ 8% of medullary carcinoma patient's basal values can be normal, providing "false-negative" results. Overall radioimmunoassays for thyrocalcitonin are established by now as extremely important tests for the diagnosis of medullary carcinoma, for the classification of familial MEN-syndromes and for the follow-up of patients after treatment for this disease.

c) Thyroglobulin Radioimmunoassay (TG)

It has already been mentioned that especially well-differentiated adeno-carcinomas of the thyroid can maintain in varying degrees the ability to trap iodide, to organify it and even to produce thyroid hormone. The substrate for organification of iodine and for thyroid hormone biosynthesis is the thyroglobulin molecule. This complex and large glycoprotein is usually confined to the interior of the thyroid cells (DeGroot, Stanbury 1975). When thyroid cell membranes are damaged, thyroglobulin is released into the circulation and then rapidly degraded by proteolytic enzymes (Dunn, Ray 1973). Therefore the molecule is not normally detectable in the serum even with sophisticated radioimmunoassays (Botsch et al. 1979). If, however, a continuous pathological process exists, which permits the release of thyroglobulin into the circulating blood, the biological degradation will not be sufficient to eliminate the protein completely and thyroglobulin concentrations can be measured by radioimmunoassays in the serum. Moderate amounts of this molecule can be detected in the blood of patients with intensive hyperplasia of the thyroid gland, with regressive changes in nodular goiters and patients with thyroiditis (Pezzino et al. 1978, Izumi, Larsen 1978). More than a decade ago it was reported, however, that thyroglobulin – often in excessive amounts – can be detected in the blood of patients with thyroid carcinoma (van Herle, Uller 1975). It was found, that thyroglobulin concentrations can increase in patients developing metastases or recurrences of thyroid cancer, even when there is no other clinical, radiological or scintigraphic evidence of such a development (Horst 1985) and therefore thyroglobuline as measured by radioimmunoassay is acknowledged today as an essential "tumor marker" to detect and follow thyroid carcinoma. From the last sentence it follows that thyroid carcinomas which lost their ability to trap iodine can still produce and release thyroglobulin (Oberdisse et al. 1980). As mentioned previously it is essential that the presence of thyroglobulin autoantibodies is ruled out, as such a situation would produce false-negative results. Methods for detecting such antibodies have been presented earlier. We do not consider the simultaneous serum analysis for autoantibodies and thyroglobulin to be essential in all serum samples. It should be performed once (usually at the first check-up after treatment of the primary lesion) and then only when clinical, radiological or scintigraphic findings suggest tumor progression and thyroglobulin remains undetectable by radioimmunoassay. Another – as yet unresolved – question is whether in "athyroid" patients after appropriate therapy of thyroid carcinoma the thyroglobulin values are valid only when substitution therapy has been withdrawn for several weeks (Reiners 1981) or whether they are valid also under administration of high thyroid hormone doses (Schatz et al. 1983). In this context it should be mentioned, that – in view of the excellent results in correlation to clinical course – thyroglobulin-RIA's were proposed several years ago as a substitute for large-dose radioiodine scans etc. in the follow-up of thyroid cancer patients (Reiners 1983) although the arguments were only partially valid (Grant et al. 1984). There were several reasons for this proposal: The patient would not have to stop thyroid hormone medication for weeks before the control-scan and would feel better subjectively, the RIA-procedure is also simpler and cheaper than other check-up studies and the patient would receive no radiation exposure. In view of the somewhat conflicting data published on this subject we are currently doing (see chapter on follow-up programs) thyroglobulin-assays in patients with thyroid carcinoma routinely on alternating conditions (once without ^{131}I-scan under thyroid hormone, once together with ^{131}I-scan after withdrawal of thyroid hormone for 1 month) during follow-up studies as described later. To our knowledge we have never missed a tumor progression with this approach in 7 years, which is much more agreeable for the patient, than the regular withdrawal of thyroid hormone one month before each check-up date. Another situation can occur, however, which is similar to the problem of the clinically bland patient with medullary thyroid carcinoma and elevated calcitonin values: namely patients with proven thyroid carcinoma in the past, high serum thyroglobulin levels and no other demonstrable signs of tumor growth. If the thyroglobulin-RIA was performed while the patient was under thyroid hormone treatment, we stop thyroid medication and recommend to do another assay together with a large-dose ^{131}I-scan after 1 month. If abnormal radioiodine uptake is found then, the therapeutic strategy is obvious (Horst 1985). If no radioiodine uptake can be detected and serum thyroglobulin remains high one must accept the fact, that thyroid carcinoma (usually of a moderately differentiated type) is growing somewhere in the patient's body and there is again the same dilemma as in calcitonin-positive patients after medullary thyroid carcinoma: Try chemotherapy or just follow the patient closely?

Case P.J., 77.23.06.27, male

January 1979: Pain in right arm, numbness in right hand. Since summer 1979 pain in both arms. Goiter known for 20 years without change. On admission (October 10th, 1979) large nodular goiter (III), firm on the right side, congestion of neck veins. On chest films phrenic nerve paresis on the right, films of spine reveal destruction of C_6 and arrosion of C_5 and C_7. Thyroid cytology suspect (Pap. III). Thyroid scan shows cold nodules. Near total thyroidectomy on October 21st, 1979, at the same intervention removal of spinal tumor masses and stabilization with palakos. Histology: Papillary thyroid cancer. Teleradiotherapy (60 Gy), 150 mCi ^{131}I on November 16th, 1979, chemotherapy (Adriamycin, Vincristine) started in March 1980 after another dose of 150 mCi ^{131}I on February 15th, 1980. October 1980: Patient without complaints, hunting(!) actively. Thyroglobulin 105 ng/ml. Situation stabilized until spring 1982 when pain was felt again in cervico-thoracic spine. ^{131}I-uptake in metastases in spine, x-ray tomography shows progressive destruction around palakos-insert. 150 mCi ^{131}I on July 23rd, 1982. Thyroglobulin 320 ng/ml. In addition 30 Gy per teleradiotherapy on spine, another 108 mCi ^{131}I on November 10th, 1982. Then significantly improved until summer 1983: Pain in left shoulder. ^{131}I-scan shows uptake in spinal lesion and in metastases in left shoulder, x-ray shows osteolytic lesion in left scapula. 100 mCi ^{131}I on August 4th, 1983, teleradiotherapy on left shoulder (40 Gy), another 100 mCi ^{131}I on December 16th, 1983. Thyroglobulin then rising to 1363 ng/ml, pain since spring 1985 worse. Orthopedic reintervention in July 1985 (tumor removal, stabilization improved, stabilization of shoulder). As total ^{131}I-dose exceeds 800 mCi chemotherapy with Aclacinomycin was started, but however still 90 mCi of ^{131}I on October 4th, 1985. Pains currently well controlled.

In a proper laboratory thyroglobulin radioimmunoassays today are not considered as technically difficult, their value for diagnosis and follow-up of thyroid carcinoma is well defined: Thyroglobulin is an excellent tumor marker especially after radical therapy of the primary thyroid carcinoma. With regard to therapeutic consequences it cannot, however, be a real substitute for radioiodine whole body scans, but it can reduce the frequency of such radionuclide in-vivo studies significantly without much danger to lose much.

Of course a variety of other substances can be produced and released especially by medullary thyroid carcinomas: thus ACTH, endorphin and biologically active amines (such as serotonin) were found in increased amounts in the sera of such patients. These phenomena, however, are not regular features of

Table 24. Tumor markers for thyroid Ca.

Marker	Normal values	Abnormal values in x types of thyroid Ca.	Consequences for management when values abnormal
CEA	< 10 ng/ml	Anaplastic Ca. Medullary Ca.	Look for sites of tumor, if positive radiotherapy, chemotherapy or surgery, if negative chemotherapy (?)
TCT (Calcitonin)	< 400 pg/ml	Medullary Ca.	Look for sites of tumor, if positive radiotherapy, surgery or chemotherapy, if negative close follow-up
TG (Thyroglobulin)	< 30 ng/ml	Adeno-Ca.	Stop hormone therapy, ^{131}I-large dose scan after 1 month. If abnormal → ^{131}I-therapy. If normal other diagnostic methods to localize tumor, possibly surgery, radiotherapy. If no tumor sites identified, close follow-up

the disease and therefore radioassays for this purpose can be considered for scientific studies only but do not form part of regular clinical diagnostic programs.

It should also be mentioned that thyroid autoantibodies – until recently detected by hemagglutination tests (see above) – can now be measured quantitatively by radioimmunoassays.

Table 24 lists normal values for the above-mentioned in vitro tests and diagnostic consequences when abnormal concentrations are found in a patient's serum.

Diagnostic Possibilities in the Future

Currently there are several trends in oncological research, which – according to preliminary results – may also provide new approaches for the diagnosis and therapeutic planning in cases with thyroid cancer. They are mostly quite sophisticated techniques which for many years will not be available for routine use in all relevant patients throughout the world.

Nuclear Magnetic Resonance Scanning

This elegant diagnostic method based on changes in the nuclear spin angles of atoms of several elements in a strong magnetic field has attracted world-wide interest in recent years for a variety of clinical studies (Hundeshagen 1984). Different magnetic resonance patterns mostly due to varying H-atom concentrations in tissue permit excellent anatomical pictures of many structures in the body (Löffler, Oppel 1981). At present the use of paramagnetic substances applied as some kind of "contrast media" is being studied to permit also the assessment of spin-echos of other atoms for clinical use (Carr et al. 1984). For lesions of the central nervous system, within the pelvis and in the heart (valves!)

the method has become clinical routine in centers in which appropriate NMR (= MRI)-systems are available (Bauer et al. 1984). Only few data, however, exist on the diagnostic potential of NMR-imaging in thyroid disease, even as it has been suggested, that such studies would be promising (Jaffiol et al. 1986). To some extent there is even an effort concerning "tissue characterization" by NMR-techniques involving perhaps also the possibility of NMR-spectroscopy (Gadian 1982). Impressive pictures of thyroid pathology have been shown (see Fig. 20) but it seems doubtful – considering the physical principles of the method – whether NMR will be able to distinguish with sufficient reliability between benign and malignant nodules in the thyroid. It certainly is an excellent technique for studying the anatomical situation in the neck and it may also be important to detect and delineate metastases of thyroid cancer in the central nervous system and it's surrounding structures. Considering the high cost of installing and operating NMR-facilities it seems doubtful – at present – whether this fascinating diagnostic approach will play a major role in diagnosis and follow-up of thyroid cancer on a broad basis in the foreseeable future. An advantage would be the lack of radiation exposure and other side effects in NMR-studies.

Immunoscintigraphy

The value of thyroglobulin-measurements in serum for the diagnosis and follow-up of thyroid carcinoma also in cases without radioiodine uptake in metastases has already been mentioned. As radioimmunoassays for thyroglobulin require a specific and potent antibody against this molecule it was evident that trials were started to label this antibody (so far mostly with ^{131}I, sometimes with ^{111}In or ^{123}I) to detect thyroglobulin-producing tumor tissue even in the absence of ^{131}I-uptake in the body (Sheperd et al. 1985). This procedure is similar to a variety of immunoscintigraphic studies in other types of neoplasms (Koch et al. 1984). With the availability of monoclonal antibodies, research was also started to assess whether certain antigen fractions would react more intensely with a specific monoclonal antibody fragment (La France et al. 1985). As in other malignancies, however, it seems that at least a combination of several monoclonal antibody fractions will be necessary to achieve a reasonably high concentration of the radiotracer in thyroid carcinomas (Fairweather et al. 1983). In view of the heterogenic morphology and pathophysiology of thyroid cancer it is no surprise that also this technique has not so far become a routine method to detect or to rule out thyroid carcinoma and it's metastases. Nevertheless it is an approach which may in the future be improved concerning diagnostic accuracy and which may lead to therapeutic applications. At present the production and purification of thyroglobulin-antibodies with high affinity in adequate amounts and their labelling with radioisotopes in a manner to provide satisfactory specific activities and sufficient count rates after in vivo application is still a problem (Schlumberger et al. 1983). As a substitute for ^{131}I, ^{123}I or ^{111}In have been proposed in immunoscintigraphic studies but these radionuclides would not allow any therapeutic applications. Readymade "kits" for labelling thyroglobulin antibodies do not yet exist therefore. For the sake of safety it would be adequate to inject a small test dose of the inactive antibody before the larger amount of labelled antibodies is given to rule out adverse reactions due to immunological phenomena. Under these circumstances immunoscintigraphy for detection of thyroid carcinoma (scans done up to 96 hrs after i.v. application of the tracer) is certainly not yet in a stage of development which would permit it's use in clinical routine studies but it does merit further interest. As soon, as the difficulties mentioned above with antibody production and labelling techniques will be overcome, the method could easily become a pillar in the framework of diagnosis of thyroid carcinoma.

Positron Emission Tomography

The method using positron emitting, mostly cyclotron produced radionuclides with frequently very short physical half-lives can – when the radioisotopes are incorporated in amino-acids or carbohydrates with increased uptake in malignant tumors – provide fascinating pictures of a variety of neoplasms (Syrota et al. 1982). The gamma-radiation resulting from the β^+-decay can be detected by two opposite detector heads or detector rings and the signals are then reconstructed by computer systems to give not only data on the activity in a certain lesion but also to permit the expression of results as the activity concentration at a given time in Bq/g and defining also the volume of the concentrating focus. Definite studies with this method on thyroid cancer are not available as yet to the author's knowledge. The costs for such diagnostic techniques would be in the same order of magnitude as those in NMR-scanning. Further research will show, if – such compounds as ^{13}N- or ^{11}C-methionin, or ^{18}F-desoxyglucose – can provide scientifically and clinically valuable results with this method in thyroid cancer. Due to the short half-lives of the radionuclides usually employed radiation exposure is almost negligible. Such studies can of course only be performed in centers in which a cyclotron unit with a radiochemical laboratory are available in the vicinity of an appropriately equipped Nuclear Medicine facility.

TSH-receptor-assays

Hormone receptor-assays in tumor tissue have gained great importance especially in the management of breast cancer (Mertz 1968). In view of all the reports on the positive effect of large thyroid hormone doses on some forms of thyroid cancer and the recently achieved possibility to measure TSH-receptors in thyroid tissue (Kohn et al. 1981) several groups started studies to find out, whether there is a correlation between the existence of TSH-receptors in thyroid carcinoma tissue and a response to suppressive thyroid hormone therapy (Edmonds, Kermode 1986). Technically such receptor-assays are much more difficult to set up than receptor-assays for steroid sex hormones, as TSH is a complex glycoprotein and in most thyroid cell membrane preparations a considerable amount of unspecific binding occurs even with purified TSH, impairing the accuracy of the assay. So far it can only be said, that – with all the inherent problems – it has been possible to develop the basic conditions for receptor assays for laboratory use. The practical clinical value of such assays for the management of thyroid cancer patients remains uncertain at present. We know that there is no correlation between receptors and ^{131}I-uptake in thyroid

Table 25a. Human tumors with receptor related defects

Group	TSH binding[a]	Glycoprotein receptor component[b]		High order gangliosides[c]		Membrane ADP ribosyltransferase activity		Membrane adenylate cyclase activity	
		Cells	Membranes			Basal	TSH-stimulated	Basal	TSH-stimulated
Non-functional thyroid tumors (9)									
I	5	Low	No	No	None	Nl	None	Nl	None
II	1	Low	No	Yes	Yes	Nl	Yes (low)	Nl	Yes (low)
III	1	Low	Modified	Modified	None	Nl	None	Nl	None
IV	1	Nl	Modified	Modified	Yes	Low	None	Low	None
V	I	Nl	Yes	Yes	Yes	Nl	Nl	Low	None
Functional thyroid tumor (1)									
	1	Nl	Yes	Yes	Above Nl G_{MI}	High	No Yes+ NAD	High Nl+ NAD	No Yes+ NAD

[a] Measured both at pH 6.0, 4 °C, and in a low salt buffer as well as at pH 7.4, 37 °C, and in 50 mM NaCl;
[b] Measured using the monoclonal antibody to the TSH receptor (43, 44);
[c] Measured by thin-layer chromatography of gangliosides from membranes sequentially exposed to periodate oxidation and sodium [^{3}H] borohydride reduction (13);
[d] Measured as ^{32}P-ADP ribose incorporation into membranes using ^{32}P-NAD as substrate (8, 17, 20, 40);
[e] Measured using the procedure of Salomon (35).

Table 25b. Parameters of TSH-receptor-binding in thyroid tumors

	Adenylate cyclase activity pmol/cAMP after 15 min/mg membrane protein	
	Normal	1-5G
Basal activity	94	782
+ TSH 1×10^{-8} M	365	840
+ NAD 1 mM	110	148
+ TSH 1×10^{-8} + NAD 1 mM	480	510

carcinoma, but we do not yet know if receptor-positive thyroid tumors are more susceptible to hormone treatment in really "suppressive" doses like estrogen-receptor-positive breast cancers, which can frequently be handled quite well with antiestrogen medication. In general it seems, that thyroid carcinoma mostly has insufficient receptor capacities in comparison with benign thyroid tissues (Table 25) and that a further differentiation of tumor characteristics and behaviour will be difficult to establish with TSH-receptor-assays only.

This last section of the chapter on diagnostic methods is meant to provide an outlook on possible future developments in the diagnosis of thyroid cancer applying the latest advances in medical technology and laboratory sciences for this purpose. It should show that the present possibilities for adequate diagnosis and follow-up of this disease – as described earlier – are already valuable but that the future may give us a variety of additional and important diagnostic approaches. It will remain the obvious duty of any concerned doctor, dealing with thyroid cancer to follow these developments and to apply them – when possible – to allow a better understanding and management of thyroid cancer.

Problems of Differential Diagnosis of Thyroid Cancer

In the clinical part of this booklet so far a variety of symptoms and other diagnostic criteria of thyroid cancer have been presented including also the most sophisticated methods available. In order to establish the clinical diagnosis of this disease in all it's various forms and with all the existing differences in the biological behaviour of the tumors the recorded data must be analyzed carefully before therapeutic strategies are worked out (Table 26). Basically therefore the most important questions for the clinician will usually be the following:

a) Under which conditions is nodular goiter probably malignant?
b) Which criteria are valid in distinguishing "thyroiditis" from thyroid cancer?
c) Under which circumstances are metastases of an unknown primary neoplasm probably of thyroid origin?

In this context it should also be mentioned that according to the literature (Shimaoka et al. 1962) about 1.5% of thyroid malignancies are not primary lesions but metastases of other cancers. Some of the most frequent and sometimes histologically puzzling secondaries in the thyroid are those hypernephroma-type renal cancers which can suggest a badly differentiated clear-cell follicular carcinoma to the reporting pathologist. Other primary tumors with metastases in the thyroid are bronchiogenic carcinoma, breast cancer, melanoma, malignant lymphoma and neoplasms of oesophagus and larynx

Table 26. Procedures for differential diagnosis in patients with suspicion of thyroid Ca.

Procedure 1	History, physical exam
Result	Suspicious nodule in thyroid, clear-cut thyroid cancer, lymph node metastases, suspicion of secondaries, Thyroiditis?
Procedure 2	Sonography, ^{99m}Tc-Scan, fine needle-biopsy, tumor markers, thyroid autoantibodies, radiological exam of chest and neck (CT, ^{201}Tl-Scan, bone scan, liver sonography)
Result	1) Thyroid cancer established (including TNM stage) 2) No convincing evidence of thyroid cancer but no definite diagnostic conclusion can be obtained 3) Thyroid cancer very unlikely

(Schwabe 1948). It was reported, that patients with a history of other cancer locations and a clinically suspicious thyroid nodule can indeed have thyroid metastases of their primary tumor in up to 5% of such cases (Abrams et al. 1950). In general, therefore, we would propose the guidelines listed Table 26 for the differential diagnosis of thyroid cancer. Stressing the clinical importance of such a diagnostic decision we would argue, that in doubtful cases the thyroid lesions should be considered as malignant as long as a careful histological study of the removed gland has not proved the contrary. In any clinically suspicious cases, however, the available diagnostic methods should be used widely to secure if possible the definite diagnosis primarily and to help in treatment planning. This approach will certainly differ in detail in developed countries and in developing countries (Riccabona 1980). Also in developing countries – perhaps stricken by endemic goiter – one should try to consider clinically suspicious nodular goiters not just as an "adaptation to iodine deficiency" (Stanbury et al. 1954), but to assess the nature of such nodular lesions possibly providing an important argument to obtain the patient's cooperation for necessary therapy. The author is well aware of the fact, that – at present – the therapeutic consequences of an exact diagnosis of thyroid cancer cannot always be realized in all parts of the world. On the other hand it must be stated, that in remote parts of our planet too one should not resign completely concerning early accurate diagnosis and adequate therapy of thyroid malignancy. The control of many other diseases in such areas has improved significantly over the past 2 decades and – as mentioned earlier – relatively few diseases can lead to such dreadful suffering and such horrible deaths as untreated thyroid cancer. With appropriate diagnostic methods at hand and relevant clinical knowledge it should be possible to minimize the death rates due to thyroid cancer in the next 2 decades all the world over.

Staging of Thyroid Cancer

With all our present diagnostic means it will frequently be possible to provide data on the spread of thyroid cancer already before primary treatment, suggesting modifications to therapeutic strategy from the beginning (Byar et al. 1979). Mostly, however, an appropriate staging of thyroid malignancies will be possible only after primary therapy (pTNM). The importance of tumor stage with regard to prognosis including also the histological classification of tumors has been discussed previously. It is important to know, that for thyroid cancer 2 staging systems currently exist:

a) TNM-classification
This – internationally accepted – classification established by the UICC (UICC 1976) has provided a system for tumor staging for all kind of malignancies. It certainly can also be applied to thyroid cancer (Gerard-Marchant 1977) and has – as shown earlier – provided important data for prognosis and therapy planning. Concerning thyroid cancer Table 27 shows the appropriate details for such classifications. On the other hand the TNM-system seemed in-

Table 27. TNM and "stage" classification of thyroid cancer

TNM a)		"Stage" b)	
T_0	"Carcinoma in situ" or no tumor detectable	I	T_0-T_1, T_2, N_0, M_0
T_1	Single lesion without invasion of surrounding structures, confined to one lobe < 1 cm Ø	II	T_0-T_2, N_0-N_2, M_0
		III	T_3, N_2, M_0
T_2	Multiple nodules, lesion confined to thyroid Ø > 1 cm	IV	T_4, N_3, M_1
T_3	Bilateral tumor confined to thyroid gland		
T_4	Tumor invasion of surrounding structures		
N_0	No lymph node metastases		
N_1	Homolateral lymph node metastases without invasion of surrounding tissue		
N_2	Bilateral or contralateral lymph node metastases		
N_3	Lymph node metastases with invasion of surrounding tissue, mediastinal lymph nodes		
M_0	No distant metastases		
M_1	Distant metastases		

adequate for a variety of malignancies, so that other staging systems were proposed also (Halnan 1982) and accepted – in part – all over the world. For thyroid cancer, trials with such more specific classification systems were started also.

b) "Stage"-classification

In view of the pecularities of thyroid cancer this staging system was proposed nearly 20 years ago (Werner 1969) dividing categories of tumor spread into 4 groups (Table 27). In some way the classification copes better with the specific growth patterns of thyroid cancer types and it can be used basically as well as the TNM-system. There are, however, "language problems" between the two systems as seen from the last table. With regard to the possibility for worldwide documentation of thyroid cancer handled by the UICC the author would therefore strongly recommend hospitals to add TNM-data to "stage"-classifications for their own files to provide comparable figures for scientific evaluation. Basically we feel, that the "stage"-system is clinically better fitted to thyroid cancer than the TNM-classification. This impression is stressed by the fact, that TNM- nomenclature has been modified several times in recent years (UICC 1979).

In conclusion therefore it can be stated that reasonable "staging"-formulae are important for prognosis and therapy of thyroid cancer. Their different "languages" should be understood world-wide and so far the TNM-system remains the "gold-standard" for studies on the spread of thyroid malignancy. Other systems need and will need an appropriate dictionary to translate their data into TNM-terms.

Therapy

As mentioned earlier therapeutic nihilism and very aggressive therapy programs were practised in cases of thyroid cancer, then histological typing of such tumors modified these approaches (Gemsenjäger 1978), so that in rather "benign" and extremely aggressive neoplasms only a minimal therapy was suggested by some authors (Taylor, Al-Wattar 1980) while other authors recommended that any type of thyroid cancer should be treated as radically as other malignancies (Clark 1982) – namely by "Stahl und Strahl" (= surgery and radiation) – and recently chemotherapy has been added to this active approach (Shimaoka 1980). When – in the following chapter – the author's opinion is presented (which was acquired during 2½ decades while handling a rather large number of thyroid cancer patients) it should be pointed out that with all the pecularities of this type of malignancy, with on-going research concerning pathogenesis and pathophysiology of these tumors (see earlier chapters) the statements made are to be seen as an "ad-hoc"-judgement of the potentials of various therapeutic strategies. Those will depend not only on scientific data, but also on a variety of factors (socio-economic, cultural, health policy) that differ very much from country to country. The primary aim, however, of any doctor confronted with the possibility of thyroid cancer in a patient must be to do everything in his power to cure a potentially fatal and terrible disease. Priorities world-wide therefore cannot only be "prescribed" in the manner of general text- books. If – e.g. – no ^{131}I-therapy and no appropriate facilities for efficient radiotherapy are available, the responsibility will mainly rest on the surgeon's capacity, which – in turn – may be restricted by local problems regarding appropriate anesthesia, hygiene, blood supply etc. Under bad conditions less may be sometimes more for the patient. On the other hand it will be shown in this chapter that an optimal combination of surgery, radiotherapy, Nuclear Medicine and oncology on the one hand with pathology on the other can sometimes provide a cure for patients with thyroid cancer, who should theoretically have died within months. As we therefore want to respect fully the individual responsibility of each doctor treating thyroid cancer, the following list of therapeutic possibilities with their results should be considered only as a reminder and a list of suggestions and not as a rule book.

1 Surgery

Many years ago a patient asked the author, whether an "atomic shot" (= ^{131}I) could not replace surgery for treatment of his thyroid cancer. Of course the answer was and will remain "no"! Surgery must be the starting point to control thyroid malignancy, regardless of advances in other therapeutic programs.

Surgery of the Primary Lesion

Except for conditions, which prohibit any surgical intervention (severe cardiac insufficiency, severe uremia, severe cerebral damage etc.) there is no situation in which some surgical approach to thyroid cancer should not be attempted. Previous diagnostic procedures will have established in many cases the individual pathology from tumor localization and spread to histological type and other important criteria such as e.g. spontaneous recurrent nerve paralysis, cardiopulmonary situation etc. These data will provide the surgeon with essential informations for his strategy and will supply answers to several questions:

a) Is there a chance of removing the tumor radically?
b) If so, will the intervention be confined to the neck or should sternotomy be considered?
c) Is the tumor growing in such an infiltrating manner, that the possitity of radical removal seems unlikely?
d) What about regional lymph nodes?
e) What about distant metastases?

ad a) What is a "radical removal" of the primary tumor?

Some groups mention, that even a local excision of the primary lesion may be adequate (Becker et al. 1984), others propose an extracapsular lobectomy of the afflicted lobe with isthmectomy (Peiper et al. 1980) in differentiated carcinomas in younger patients, some demand "total thyroidectomies" and still another group feels that "near-total thyroidectomy" (Lobectomy on the afflicted side and subtotal resection of the contralateral lobe) should be practised (Esselstyn 1983). As we know from long-term follow-up studies and from histological reports (Iida et al. 1969) a procedure limited only to the afflicted lobe involves a greater risk of recurrences (Tollefsen et al. 1972). On the other hand radical total thyroidectomies carry a relatively high risk of postoperative complications such as recurrent nerve damage and tetany (Table 28). Between too little and too much we have fared well for many years with "near-total thyroidectomies" (see above) when thyroid cancer was suspected. The complication rate is acceptable (Table 28) and the rate of local recurrences remains low (< 10%). This approach is also carried out in recurrent goiters, if there is no previous recurrent nerve lesion on the contralateral side of the tumor. If such a situation should exist, however, an intracapsular removal of the tumor may be considered. The question of a proper identification of recurrent larnygeal nerves (Edis et al. 1975) and at least 2 parathyroid glands (Attie, Khafif 1975)

Table 28. Complications after surgery for thyroid cancer

	Oberdisse, Klein, Reinwein	Own material	Winter et al. 1986
Mortality	5.6%	0.3%	0.6%
Unilateral rec. nerve paralysis	~15.0%	10.0%	2.5%
Bilateral rec. nerve paralysis	~15.0%	0.4%	0.2%
Tetany	~ 1.7%	1.0%	25.0%
Tracheostomy	2.0%	0.5%	0.2%
Other	~ 8.0%	1.0%	2.4%

has been discussed extensively. We certainly agree with dissecting the recurrent laryngeal nerve free on the side of a planned extracapsular lobectomy, but identification of the nerve "by palpation" is sometimes adequate and in some patients after all the accurate preparation of the nerve you will be in a situation in which you can either preserve the nerve and risk remainders of tumor tissue or sacrifice the nerve for the sake of a really radical operation. If the contralateral recurrent nerve is regular we certainly would recommend sacrificing the nerve and removing the neoplasm entirely under such circumstances. Modern logopedic methods (Boehme 1983), sometimes helped by strychnine injections (20 mg N-Oxyde-Strychnine-Diethylaminoethanol daily for 2 weeks) frequently reduce the phonetic consequences of unilateral recurrent nerve lesions (Riccabona 1973) and in many cases (35%) recurrent nerve damage exists for only a few months and normal vocal chord function can return afterwards.

Case K.B., female, 49.02.04.65

In 1982 lymph nodes in the neck, proposed biopsy rejected. Since 1984 pain in neck, palpitation, nervousness. Exam (elsewhere) reveals multiple large lymph-nodes on both sides of the neck and nodular goiter, chest films regular, cold thyroid nodules, lymph-nodes also cold, cytology Pap. IV. Intervention under the assumption of thyroid cancer on September 13th, 1985: near total thyroidectomy with removal of lymph-nodes on the left (elsewhere). Histology: papillary Ca. with lymph-node metastases. Postoperatively bilateral vocal chord paralysis, hypocalcemia. Admission on October 11th, 1985: large palpable tumor masses on the left neck side. Thyroglobulin 75 ng/ml, bilateral vocal chord paralysis, calcium 2.08 mmol/l, BSR 9/20, on scan ^{131}I-uptake in nodules in the neck. Modified neck dissection on the left on October 15th, 1985 with macroscopically radical removal of lymph-node metastases. Telecurietherapy (40 Gy), 100 mCi ^{131}I on October 25th, 1985. Upon discharge calcium normal with Vitamin D_3 and calcium, *normal* vocal chord mobility on the right, left vocal chord still paralytic.

If vocal chord function does not return a variety of surgical procedures exists (Naumann 1972) which can provide adequate phonetics and respiration. Details of the technique of recurrent nerve dissection are given in the surgical literature (Fuchsig, Keminger 1972) including microscopic methods. The large number of anatomical variants in the course of the recurrent laryngeal nerve

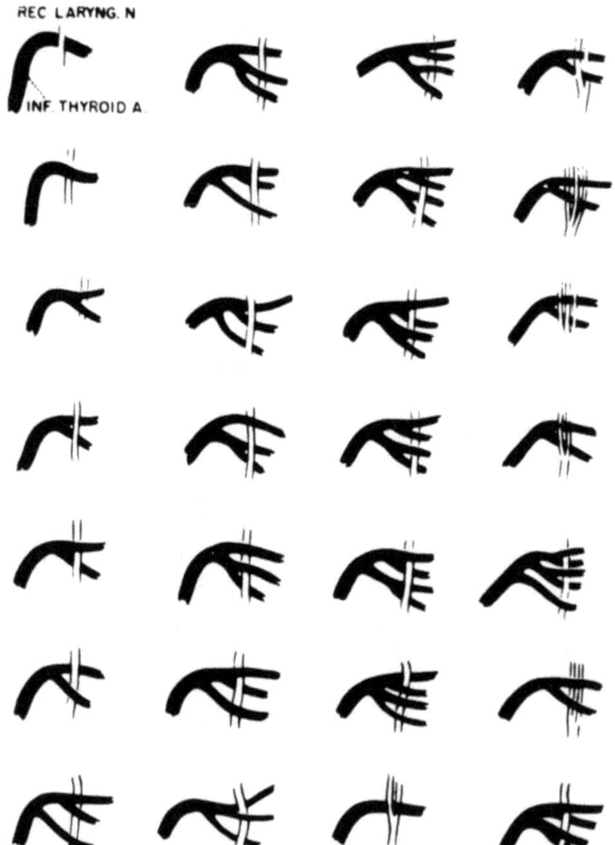

Fig. 37. Anatomical variations of recurrent laryngeal nerve in relation to inferior thyroid artery

(Fig. 37) should be known so as to be able to look for the nerve in the right place. With regard to the identification and preservation of parathyroid glands the author has had the experience that tetany was most common in surgical services in which these procedures were carried out meticulously. The dissecting of normal parathyroids is bound to produce frequently vascular damage to these glands (Thompson et al. 1973) impairing their function. If a parathyroid gland is seen, it can either be preserved or implanted in arm muscles (Hickey, Samaan 1975), but the preservation of these small structures should never inhibit radical tumor surgery. As hypoparathyroidism can be controlled adequately by Vitamin D or Tachyhydrosterol (AT 10) and Calcium (Becker et al. 1984), hypocalcemia cannot be considered as a very serious complication after radical surgery of a malignant tumor. It must also be mentioned that regeneration of perhaps one remaining parathyroid gland is responsible for the fact that almost 50% of postoperative tetanic symptoms will be transient (see Table 29).

Another problem involves the cases in which thyroid malignancy is detected only postoperatively after a routine thyroid resection due to careful histological examination of the specimen (Huber, Riccabona 1967). Can routine "frozen

Table 29. Transient and permanent complications after surgery for thyroid cancer

	Total	Transient	Permanent
Recurrent nerve paralysis	10.4%	3.80%	6.24%
Tetany	1.0%	0.66%	0.34%

sections" prevent such awkward situations? Should reinterventions after such histology reports always be done?

In the author's personal experience – which is probably influenced by his training in pathology – a careful macroscopic inspection of a removed thyroid can be as valuable as an intraoperative "frozen section" or an "instant imprint histology" with a diagnostic accuracy of ~93% (Suen et al. 1978). Even in collaboration with experienced pathologists it is possible to obtain a malignant final classification perhaps 1 week after the intervention from a specimen which was considered as benign in the "frozen section". This is due to the fact, that only careful slice-by-slice examination of the removed thyroid can sometimes provide adequate evidence for the definite diagnosis as mentioned earlier (Cabanne et al. 1974). In clinically suspicious nodules we would therefore recommend to choose a surgical approach as if malignancy were proven on the afflicted side, inspecting and cutting the specimen and to obtain a "frozen section". Macroscopic criteria of thyroid cancer are well described in pathology textbooks (Fassbender 1956): Firm, solid, whitish lesions with little colloid especially with unclear delineation to the surrounding parenchyma as well as whitish lesions with necrotic masses in the center and proliferating tissue around the necrosis are suspicious of thyroid cancer even when there is no invasion of surrounding structures. The same conclusions can be drawn from cystic lesions with papillary tumors in their wall. It can also help if the typical neck lymphpathways are explored at the primary intervention (see later). If lymph nodes resembling "aberrant thyroid tissue" are found, the diagnosis of thyroid cancer is certain (King, Pemberton 1942). It was stated earlier, that e.g. "hot" or "warm" nodules are malignant in only relatively few cases and that cytology and sonography provide further informations on the nature of thyroid nodules. Even though this remains true, none of the techniques mentioned is as informative as a careful look at *any* exposed and/or removed thyroid by an experienced surgeon's eye and a *"representative"* frozen section examined by an equally experienced pathologist to establish a correct diagnosis at the best time (Schauer 1984). The answer to the second question (reintervention?) is easier to give when the guidelines of question 1 mentioned in the respective answers are respected. The situation of malignancy reported only days or weeks after the primary intervention, however, can occur even in centers with optimal diagnostic facilities and experienced staff in surgery and pathology. In general "microcarcinomas" with a diameter of less than 1,5 cm diameter and a differentiated histological tumor pattern can be considered as "radically" removed if there is no evidence of lymph-node metastases and if the tumor does not infiltrate the margin of the specimen. On the other hand it should be known, that also small primary lesions can produce massive lymph node secondaries:

Case F.B., female, 24.23.09.64

Since summer 1979 growth of lymph node on right neck side. Biopsy (elsewhere) in November 1979: Metastasis of papillary thyroid Ca. No history of irradiation during childhood. On admission irregular shaped, tender, firm thyroid nodule on the right, extrathyroidal tumor in the right just above the sternal notch. Multiple enlarged and firm lymph nodes on the left. Near total thyroidectomy with neck dissection on the right and modified neck dissection on the left on December 12th, 1979. Histology: Papillary thyroid Ca. (multicentric) with bilateral lymph node metasases. Teleradiotherapy (60 Gy), 100 mCi ^{131}I on January 4th, 1982. Patient then doing well until May 1982: lymph node on right neck side. Removal on June 3rd, 1982: Metastasis. Since then patient doing well, thyroglobulin normal, no evidence of metastases or recurrence, with thyroid hormone studies continued successfully.

Finally – especially if the guidelines mentioned above are neglected – cases occur in which thyroid surgery for hyperthyroidism or non-toxic nodular goiter is carried out on a routine basis and the pathology reveals a malignant thyroid tumor either of more than 1.5 cm diameter or involving both lobes (Nishiyama et al. 1977). In cases with "microtumors" (= minimal thyroid carcinoma") of differentiated carcinomas without evidence of metastases we do not think that a reintervention would be necessary with all it's increased risks for the recurrent laryngeal nerves (Huber, Riccabona 1967), which are sometimes difficult to identify in fresh, hyperemic and friable scar tissue (Taylor et al. 1976). On the other hand it seems essential, that in larger tumors detected "by chance", in bilateral tumor foci and in cases with positive lymph nodes reinterventions should be done as early as possible, especially if the tumor is undifferentiated (Table 30). The "reintervention" will usually include the total removal of the thyroid remnant on the afflicted side and a subtotal removal of the contralateral lobe as well as a lymph node exploration (Riccabona 1986). As mentioned above, the risk of recurrent nerve damage and other local complications increases significantly in such procedures, but the better long-term results (Oberdisse et al. 1980) certainly justify such an aggressive therapy. In this context we would like to remind all surgeons that specimens of each thyroid lobe should either be packed for the pathologist in separately labeled bags or that – e.g. – the specimen of the right lobe should be marked with a thread. Identification of the afflicted lobe becomes easy by such simple methods and can help to plan an eventual reintervention, which in general should be performed by the surgeon who did the first procedure.

Table 30. Indications for reintervention after surgery of thyroid Ca. (after regular thyroid surgery)

1st)	Histology report shows multicentric Ca. or invasion of specimen border by Ca.
2nd)	Histology report shows poorly differentiated or anaplastic Ca.
3rd)	Histology report shows tumor of > 1.5 cm diameter
4th)	Histology report shows lymph node involvement

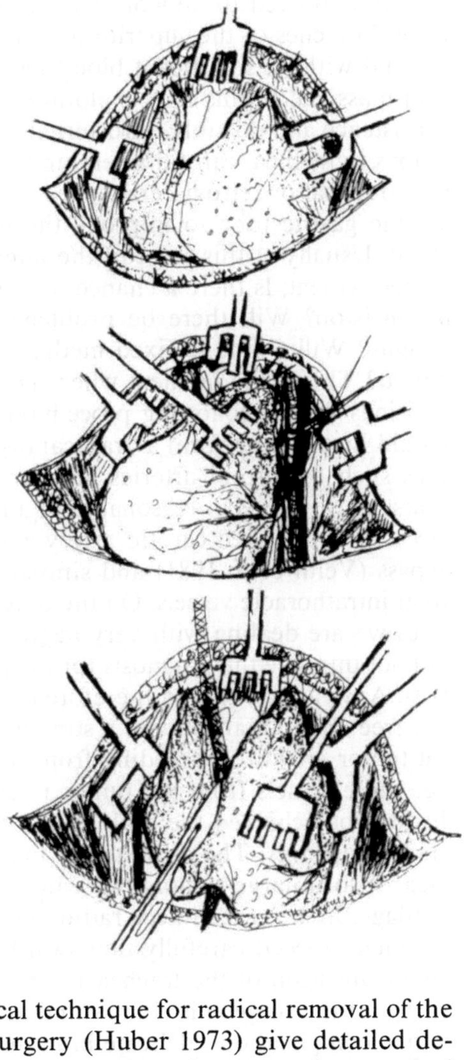

Fig. 38. *Above:* exposure of thyroid tumor on the left: after collar incision neck veins are cut after being tied, straight neck muscles are separated in the midline and cut transversely on side of the tumor. Appropriate skin-platysma flaps provide sufficient access to thyroid gland.
Middle: branches of superior thyroid artery have been tied and cut to mobilize the upper pole of the left thyroid lobe, traction is applied to the left lobe after it was dissected free and the important anatomical structures are identified and marked with straps (iugular vein, carotid artery, vagal and recurrent laryngeal nerve), parathyroids are identified. Dissection of tumor in relation to these structures.
Below: after the tumor was cleared from vessels and nerves the thyroid isthmus is cut on a Kocher type sonde and the trachea is dissected free. After these manoeuvres the tumor bearing lobe can be removed in toto

Let us now consider the typical surgical technique for radical removal of the primary thyroid cancer. Textbooks of surgery (Huber 1973) give detailed descriptions of the classical approach. It is not common, however, that atypical anatomical situations are described as well and that appropriate advice is given. In cases without neck nodes a typical transverse collar incision through the platysma is made under general anesthesia with orotracheal intubation. Neck veins are ligated, superior and inferior skin-platysma flaps are dissected free, giving an access from the hyoid bone to the dorsal surface of the sternal notch (Fig. 38). Cervical strap muscles are separated in the midline and can be cut transversely, when large lesions exist. If they are infiltrated by tumor the respective muscle parts are left with the tumor and further exposure of the thyroid should be carried out through healthy muscles. If possible we then try to dissect free a tissue layer covering normal thyroid parenchyma (capsula thyreoidea propria). In large lesions this procedure can take time and needs patience. In many cases, however, which were primarily considered as "inoperable" the effort proved to be worthwhile: Once the surgeon arrives in such a tissue layer, branches of the superior and inferior thyroid arteries can be ligated and cut and without significant blood loss a further digital exploration of the thyroid mass can begin. This exploration should provide information on the size, consistence and possibly retrosternal growth of the tumor, it's topographical relations to trachea, carotid artery and oesophagus. In cases with widening of the retrotracheal or retrovisceral spaces on radiographs we therefore usually insert a large gastric tube to improve the identification of the oesophagus (Huber 1973). Usually at this stage of the intervention the further surgical strategy becomes evident: Is there a chance of removing the tumor radically from the collar incision? Will there be problems with carotid arteries, trachea or oesophagus? Will – due to fixed mediastinal tumor masses – a sternotomy be required? This is the moment when the surgeon has to make the most important decisions for the following procedure! He should not resign too easily but nor should he try to perform a "radical thyreoidectomy" in cases in which vital organs such as carotid arteries and large vessels in the chest are involved. Of course it would seem reasonable in an era of advanced vascular surgery to resect a tumor-packed carotid artery and restore blood flow to the brain with a bypass (Veith et al. 1981) and similar approaches seem also possible with the great intrathoracic vessels. On the other hand we should not forget that in such cases we are dealing with very aggressive cancers and vascular reconstruction will not improve the prognosis for the patient significantly when such situations exist. Anyway one should therefore try in large tumors to dissect the carotid artery free and to mark it with a strap as well as the jugular vein in an area without tumor growth. Proceeding from this mark it will frequently be possible to free these vessels from the tumor in careful blunt and sharp dissection and if this can be achieved the outlook for a successful radical operation of thyroid cancer improves. The next step is the identification and dissection of the trachea. Also in large tumors one can usually free the upper part of the thyroid cartilage. In the case of neck radiographs showing deviations of the trachea one can then proceed carefully downwards along the anterior wall of the trachea. Tumor invasion of the trachea in this region can produce large lesions in the trachea if the surgeon is clumsy and as such lesions can provoke severe postoperative complications, delicate blunt manoeuvres are recommended to identify the thyroid gland's isthmus which can then be split, so that the anterior tracheal wall is freed. At this stage you should have the tumor mass freed from the large neck vessels and the anterior tracheal wall. If no fixed mediastinal masses exist – which would require sternotomy – lateral vessels around the tumor are ligated and cut beginning from the front of the lesion, the recurrent nerve is identified at the site where it crosses the inferior thyroid artery and the afflicted lobe is gradually lifted up. Keeping away from the recurrent nerve it is gradually removed by blunt and sharp manoeuvres from the trachea and (on the left side) from the oesophagus, while still some small vessels must be ligated and cut. During this phase of the procedure one can sometimes observe that firm, white tissue layers remain on the walls of the trachea, larynx or oesophagus. We would certainly not recommend to remove them by force thus producing defects in the trachea etc., which would produce a variety of complications.

In cases in which it is impossible to free the carotid artery from the tumor we still recommend to leave tumor tissue around the artery, to resect – if necessary – the jugular vein and to remove as much of the tumor as possible. When tumor masses fill the jugular vein at the inferior resection edge one can try to remove them by suction.

On the other hand, surgical strategy has to be changed if intrathoracic tumor masses exist (Sedgwick 1974). We would warn against making any forced efforts to remove such tumor parts from the neck in a manoeuvre which can end tragically (Huber 1973). In these patients a typical sternotomy should be performed together with the collar incision right from the beginning. Depending on the location of the intrathoracic thyroid cancer, thoracotomy can sometimes provide a better access to the tumor than sternotomy. The great vessels in the anterior mediastinum are then identified and marked by straps (Fig. 39) and the surgeon will then try to remove the intrathoracic tumor parts by blunt and sharp dissection, sparing the vessels and – deeper inside the chest – trachea and bronchial bifurcation. Invasion of the pericardium can sometimes be found and – if possible – these infiltrated parts of pericardium can be resected, together with the tumor. In a few cases even resections of the right atrial wall were performed successfully to remove intrathoracic thyroid cancer in toto. Care should be applied to detect pleural lesions in time and to handle them appropriately. Adequate drainage of course is mandatory after all such interventions. Facilities for adequate postoperative care must be available in all hospitals in which such procedures are performed and an adequate supply of blood units is mandatory.

Even as it was said, that in cases with tumor invasion of the trachea and larynx one should – in general – rather leave some tumor tissue with these structures, there are a few cases in which laryngectomy or tracheal resection should at least be considered (Riccabona 1986): In patients with differentiated

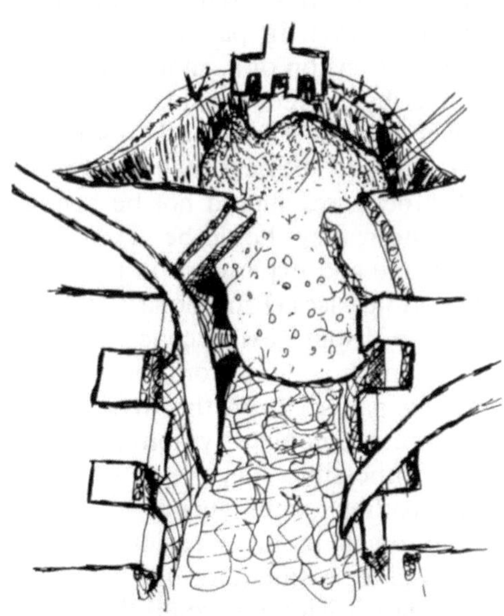

Fig. 39. Access by sternotomy to endothoracic thyroid Ca. Tumor of the *left* thyroid lobe reaching down to the pericardium, left carotid artery and iugular vein secured, *right* subclavian and pulmonary vessels are also secured. Next step would be to dissect the left subclavian vessels, left pulmonary vessels and the aortic arch

carcinoma and a localized intratracheal or endolaryngeal tumor growth leading to severe respiratory distress and without other metastases it should be realized that we can cure such cases with such radical interventions, whereas they will otherwise die after palliative tracheostomy and a long terrible suffering:

Case W.M., female, 94.01.05.19

Growth of recurrent goiter in 1967 with increasing dyspnoea and hoarseness. At first exam in November 1967 large, firm and only partially mobile nodular recurrent goiter (right > left), nodules mostly cold, recurrent nerve paralysis on the right, severe tracheal compression on radiograms of neck. Near-total thyroidectomy on November 11th, 1967 (unradical because of invasion of the trachea). Histology: Follicular carcinoma with moderate differentiation. In chest films postoperatively metastases in upper lung on the right. 90 mCi ^{131}I on December 1st, 1967, radiotherapy (~40 Gy), another 90 mCi ^{131}I on March 1st, 1968. Doing well until June 1970: Then increasing respiratory distress, no palpable recurrence, chest film regular, endoscopy shows subglottic endolaryngeal tumor. Therefore laryngectomy on June 30th, 1970. Having learned to talk again, doing well, no metastases, no recurrence until spring 1972: ^{131}I-uptake in right lung: 120 mCi ^{131}I, remission until 1974. Again uptake in the right lung, 120 mCi ^{131}I on February 2nd, 1974 and on May 16th, 1974. Since then doing well, no evidence of recurrence or metastases, no thyroglobulin detectable in serum.

After obtaining the informed consent of such a patient we would suggest to remove the primary lesion as mentioned and then – with trachea and larynx free – to proceed with a classical laryngectomy (Naumann 1972) or with tracheal resection (Beall et al. 1962). The latter procedure is definitely more of a problem: In the neck the end-to-end anastomosis after circumferential resection is a problem per se (Barclay et al. 1957) and may end in severe strictures after some time even in patients with normal postoperative course. On the other hand the excision of a smaller portion of the tracheal wall (e.g. anterolaterally) covered by a free transplant of nasal septum and mucosa or rib cartilage (Meyer 1971) will frequently not provide as radical a cure than circumferential resections and stillbear the risk of postoperative stenosis (Grillo 1968). Anyway such procedures should not be considered routine in the management of thyroid cancer, they should be planned carefully by a surgical team with adequate knowledge and experience in these techniques and remain restricted to only a few eligible cases (Riccabona 1986).

Some dispute exists concerning the extent and technical modalities of regional lymph node exploration during the primary intervention. The lymphatic draining pattern from the thyroid gland is complex (Spiessl et al. 1982) and therefore a complete lymph-node exploration from a regular collar incision seems impossible. On the other hand the most frequently afflicted cervical nodes leading to and lying along the jugular vein can very well be explored with this approach. As an extension of the primary incision as for modified neck dissection gives cosmetic results which certainly are less favourable than the normal collar incision we would therefore recommend to rely primarily on the collar incision. After removal of the cervical tumor, the jugular vein should be identified from just below the mandibular angle down to the sternoclavicular joint. Then the soft tissues around the vein between trachea and jugular vein and below the inferior pole of the thyroid lobes should be explored – perhaps using magnification – and lymph nodes should be removed and sent to the pathologist for frozen-section studies. Of course the approach has to be different when lymph node metastases are known clinically and the surgical strategy to be applied in such cases will be described later. At the end of such an intervention to remove the primary thyroid tumor the surgeon will have to classify his work: Was the procedure radical (T_0-T_3, N_1-N_2) or did he leave tumor tissue in the body (T_4, N_3, M_1)? This will be important to facilitate further therapy planning! One can also mark residual tumor areas with clips to provide exact information for radiotherapy planning. After difficult interventions the orotracheal tube should be removed while still in the operating room to check, if the patient is breathing regularly. In case of respiratory distress (recurrent nerve damage, intratracheal tumor growth), do not hesitate to perform a tracheostomy – which frequently can be closed later – to avoid hypoxemia in the postoperative period (Huber, Riccabona 1967).

Extensive surgery for thyroid cancer such as described here will – of course – be accompanied by a higher rate of complications than in regular thyroid interventions (see above). Moreover patients are left functionally "athyroid" or "hypothyroid" and require lifelong thyroid hormone medication. These were the reasons, why several surgeons proposed much less radical procedures for thyroid cancer in "low-risk-groups" (well-differentiated papillary carcinoma, young patients, T_0-T_2) (Becker et al. 1984), suggesting that lobectomies of the afflicted side and isthmectomies would be perfectly adequate to control the disease. We know that such tumors can show a relapse after decades, and we know that they can change their biological behaviour and that they frequently occur bilaterally (see above). So it seems justified to insist on bilateral more or less radical procedures as described previously, where there is no "microcarcinoma" detected by chance just as we would not recommend total extracapsular thyroidectomy with "prophylactic" neck-dissections on the other hand in any thyroid cancer case (Horst 1985). We should provide a human, serious and

Table 31. Results of surgery (combined with other therapeutic methods) in radically operated patients and in patients with palliative surgery only

		5 yr. survival		10 yr. survival	
		Endemic area (Austria)	Goiter free zone (Japan)	Endemic area (Austria)	Goiter free zone (Japan)
Radical operations	T_{0-3}	75.0%	99.0%	61.0%	73.8%
	N_{0-2}	58.2%	91.5%	34.7%	86.0%
	M_0	/	/	/	/
Palliative surgery	T_4	21.4%	60.0%	0.5%	21.4%
	N_3	29.4%	46.5%	17.3%	43.0%
	M_1	25.5%	25.0%	8.0%	15.0%

well-balanced surgical strategy for thyroid cancer, whenever we are aware, that "too little" will leave patient and doctor in a possibly awkward situation many years later and that "too much" can be an almost crippling experience for the patient. In the complex therapy pattern of thyroid cancer the role of surgery per se is difficult to assess. The essential benefits of appropriate surgery, however, can be deducted from statistics showing the high rate of definite cures in surgically treatable cases (T_0-T_3, N_0-N_2) in comparison with groups in which the surgeon could not remove all tumor masses (T_4, N_3, M_1): Table 31.

Surgery of Metastases

Surgery of Lymph Node Metastases

In this context I shall not talk about those cases, in which cervical lymph nodes removed by chance reveal the existence of metastases of thyroid cancer: In that event the cure of the primary tumor as mentioned previously will be the next step in surgical therapy. Instead I will focus on those patients who present clinically obvious lymph node metastases of thyroid cancer right from the beginning:

Case D'A.G., female, 02.05.08.70

No history of irradiation in childhood. Since January 1983 nervousness, feeling tired. Thyroid exam (elsewhere): "Thyroiditis". Medical treatment provides transient improvement. Since July 1984 growth of lateral neck mass on the right. Subtotal thyroidectomy on December 28th, 1984 (elsewhere). Histology: Papillary Ca. On admission (January 20th, 1985) multiple large lymph nodes on the right neck side. Sonography shows impression of right jugular vein, chest film regular, on ^{131}I-scan only uptake in small thyroid remnants. Modified neck-dissection on the right with resection of jugular vein on January 21st, 1985. Teleradiotherapy (60 Gy), 50 mCi ^{131}I on February 15th, 1985. In May 1985 swelling in right submandibular angle. Sonography shows nodule at the upper angle of the scar on the right with reduced echos, ^{131}I-scan shows uptake in this area. 147 mCi ^{131}I on May 25th, 1985. Reintervention on June 16th, 1985 with removal of partially necrotic lymph node metastases on the right. Thyroglobulin now 29 ng/ml, diffuse swelling of right parotid gland, no evidence of tumor or metastases by scan, radiographs, sonography and clinically, no complaints.

The removal of the primary lesion is mandatory and then the afflicted lymph nodes should be cleared as well. Primarily our strategy remains a "modified neck dissection" (Edis et al. 1975) in these cases, although depending on the anatomical situations we sometimes end up with a classical "radical neck dissection" (Keminger 1964). Anyway the collar incision for removal of the primary tumor is extended upwards along the anterior border of the sternocleidomastoid muscle to the mandibular angle and downwards to the sternoclavicular joint of the afflicted side. Depending on the site of pathological lymph nodes it may also be drawn into the submandibular triangle and in the supraclavicular fossa. After securing the jugular veins and carotid arteries we proceed as mentioned in the section on lymph node exploration during surgery of the primary tumor. The wider access, however, provides better possibilities to remove even large lymph node masses. The vagal and phrenic nerves are preserved, care should be taken to avoid lesions of the thoracic duct when operating on the left side and at the end of the procedure the whole space between cervical spine, trachea, larynx and submandibular salivary gland and upper thoracic aperture should be cleared, leaving only carotid arteries and the mentioned nerves in place. When the submandibular triangle is explored the inferior branch of the facial nerve should be spared and not damaged by traction or direct trauma, while the submandibular gland can be sacrificed. Dissecting free lymph nodes located high up in the neck and just before the cervical spine may cause problems with preservation of the accessory nerve and the cervical plexus, while in dorsal parts of the lower neck the brachial plexus should also be spared. In cases of bilateral lymph node involvement, resections or ligation of both jugular veins should be avoided, as severe congestion in the head can occur after such procedures (Huber 1973). As mentioned earlier it may be appropriate in some cases to remove the sternocleidomastoid muscle, cutting it at it's sternoclavicular insertion and then gradually mobilizing it upwards until it is severed below the base of the skull. This leaves the patient with a real deformation of the neck, usually with litte functional disturbance but makes it possible to remove large lymph node masses more radically, leaving sternocleidomastoid fibers attached to the tumor and resecting the whole mass "en bloc". Interventions for lymph node metastases of thyroid cancer can therefore start as extended lymph node explorations becoming modified neck dissections and even classical radical neck dissections depending on the anatomical situation. Anyway the goal of these procedures should be to reduce a $T_{0-3}/N_1-N_2/M_0$ stage to a $T_0/N_0/M_0$ situation without severe consequences for the patient (Table 32). Reinterventions for similar purposes are justified but as a careful dissection in scar tissue is technically much more difficult than at a primary intervention and macroscopic evaluation of tissue is also a problem sometimes, the practical considerations will sometimes limit the radicality of such procedures, as long as the principle of "primum nil nocere" prevails.

Surgery of distant metastases of thyroid cancer

The current surgical possibilities for the elimination of distant metastases of thyroid cancer using bone replacement, orthopedic stabilization, and the tech-

Table 32. Complications after radical neck dissection

	Oberdisse, Klein, Reinwein n=~110	Own material n=23
Mortality	2.7%	4.6%
Recurrent nerve paralysis	20.4%	25.0%
Tetany	2.0%	/
Other	8.2%	4.6%

niques of modern neurosurgeons and thoracic surgeons seem to be almost without limits. On the other hand we must be aware of the fact that surgeons are dealing in such situations with a malignant disease which has possibly spread throughout the body. The removal of a secondary lesion will therefore only be justified where no other adequate possibility for treatment exists, where a well-defined lesion is responsible for serious symptoms or where there is satisfactory evidence that the metastasis to be removed really is a solitary lesion (Riccabona 1986). Under these circumstances surgery can be considered as a very efficient therapeutic possibility in the management of metastatic thyroid cancer (Riccabona 1977) (Table 33). Perhaps the most fascinating successes were reported from orthopedic surgeons in recent years (Roy Camille et al. 1986), who are able today to remove bone metastases in spine, pelvis and limbs with adequate stabilization (Fig. 40). Taking into account the frequently slow growth of differentiated thyroid carcinomas such interventions may also provide long-term relief for patients with other metastases (see case P. J., p. 87):

Even if these patients will not be "tumor-free" after the orthopedic correction of a bone metastasis they can for many years live without pain and no mobility problems. Otherwise we would strictly prefer surgical removal of a single brain metastasis where technically feasible to radioiodine treatment of such lesions: We know cases which developed severe edema and hemorrhage in cerebral secondaries with high radioiodine uptake after therapy and even died due to these complications:

Case Z.H., 99.12.04.34, female

1969 subtotal thyroidectomy elsewhere: histologically "papillary structures", but no evidence of cancer. In 1977 growth of a tumor on the head, surgery on

Table 33. Results of surgery for metastases of thyroid cancer

Type of intervention	No. of cases	Results
Tracheoplasty after tracheal resection	1	
Chordotomy	7	
Laryngectomy	2	mean survival time 38.7 months
Lung resections	2	
Cervical spine resection and fusion	3	20% actually $T_0M_0N_0$
Removal of soft tissue metastases and recurrent lymph nodes	17	40% actually living
Joint resection and endoprothesis	3	15% deceased not due to thyroid cancer
Hemilaminectomy	7	
Removal of cerebral metastases	2	45% deceased due to thyroid cancer
Bone resections	7	
(Tracheostomy)	(8)	
(Gastrostomy)	(2)	
Total: ( ) = emergency procedures	51 (61)	

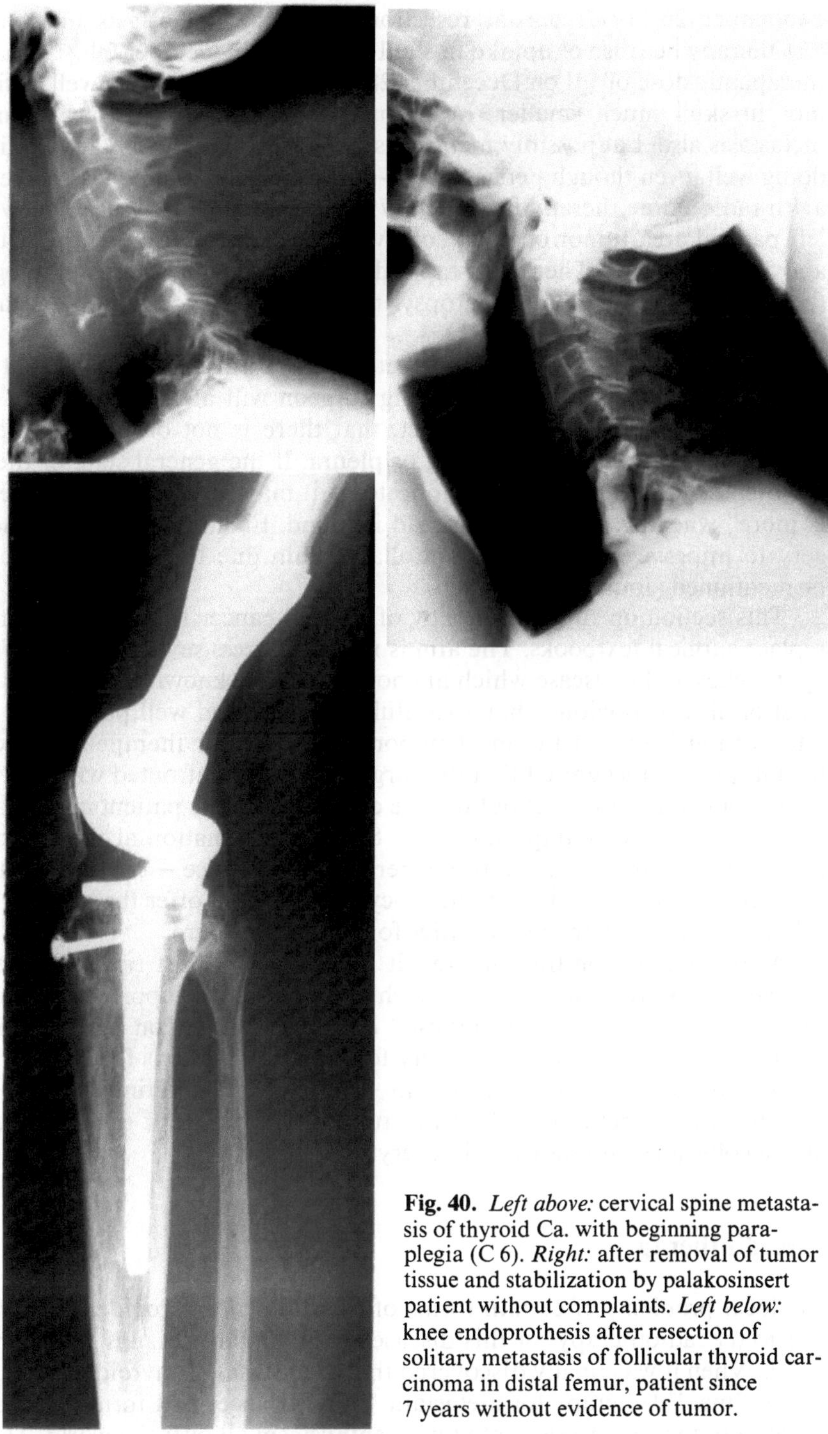

Fig. 40. *Left above:* cervical spine metastasis of thyroid Ca. with beginning paraplegia (C 6). *Right:* after removal of tumor tissue and stabilization by palakosinsert patient without complaints. *Left below:* knee endoprothesis after resection of solitary metastasis of follicular thyroid carcinoma in distal femur, patient since 7 years without evidence of tumor.

September 26, 1977: partial resection, histology: metastasis of thyroid Ca. ^{131} I-therapy because of uptake in skull and chest on October 7th, 1977. Another therapeutic dose of ^{131}I on December 28th, 1977. Patient doing well, residual tumor in skull much smaller. In August 1978 skull focus nearly gone, chest metastasis also, but possibly metastasis in sacrum. 3rd ^{131}I-therapy. Patient then doing well, even though persistent ^{131}I-uptake in skull and pelvis was reason for a 4th radioiodine therapy in April 1979. In September 1979 besides swelling in left parotid area tumor on skull somewhat larger, teleradiotherapy with 40 Gy and 5th ^{131}I-therapy. Thereafter rapid deterioration with severe neurological defects, death after 1 month. Autopsy: necrotic skull and brain metastasis with hemorrhage into ventricles.

Easily accessible solitary lung metastases can also be excised, but even in the age of CT-scanning the exploring surgeon will after opening the chest be confronted sometimes with the fact, that there is not only the one expected lesion but multiple lesions in lung or pleura. If the general state of the patient permits in such circumstances a lobectomy it may be done, but in general "less is more" when a wider tumor spread is found. Finally the scope for neurosurgery to improve otherwise uncontrollable pain due to metastases should also be mentioned (Joumans 1982).

This section on surgical therapy of thyroid cancer is certainly not meant to replace surgical textbooks. The aim is rather to stress several aspects of surgical approaches to the disease which are not adequately known in many institutions. First of all it is obvious, that a carefully planned and well performed primary intervention is one of the most important factors for therapeutic success and then it must be recognised that the surgeon will be confronted with thyroid cancer not only after it's onset but that he can also help the patient in later stages of the disease in a very important way. Surgical resignation at the beginning on the other hand is – in the author's personal experience – one of the most serious errors in dealing with a malignancy which would offer through it's biological pecularities so many possibilities for a long-time cure.

A final remark on this chapter: It is certainly against established ethics in the medical profession if a surgeon who has neither the appropriate training or suitable facilities and has recognised centers in his region decides on radical surgery for thyroid cancer or surgery for metastatic lesions for his own benefit. It am convinced that a surgeon who – instead of operating himself – refers such patients to better qualified institutions will be better off in the long run, than a colleague who wants to do everything himself.

2 Radiotherapy

The local problems of certain forms of thyroid cancer provided plenty of reasons to try radiotherapy for this disease already many decades ago (Pemberton 1939). When it was finally discovered that metastases of thyroid cancer can trap radioiodine, ^{131}I-therapy for metastatic thyroid cancer as a form of selective internal radiotherapy was accepted with enthusiasm all over the world. The possibility of treating pleural effusions due to metastases of thyroid cancer with radioactive colloids further improved the scope of radiotherapy of this disease (Seidlin et al. 1949). With the description of labeled thyroglobulin antibodies concentrated in thyroid malignancies a further approach in isotope therapy for thyroid cancer seems to have become possible as mentioned previously. Therefore the various forms of radiotherapy must be considered as an essential part of the treatment of thyroid cancer and the various applications under individual circumstances will be discussed in the following chapter.

Teleradiotherapy

Teleradiotherapy on the Neck

In past decades conventional x-ray therapy was frequently applied with a varying success rate in cases in which the primary tumor was classified as inoperable by surgeons (Steiner, Salis-Samaden 1966). In some cases a palliation effect could be observed for months and years (Portmann 1941). If, when and how teleradiotherapy should be used, however, after surgery of thyroid cancer (just as postoperative radiotherapy is used after breast cancer surgery) is still an open question (Oberdisse et al. 1980). We certainly are convinced that this kind of treatment should be applied to all "high-risk-group"-patients with thyroid cancer routinely (badly differentiated carcinomas and/or sarcomas, T_3-T_4/N_2-N_3-stages and patients above 45 years) (Horst 1985). The reason for this rather aggressive attitude is the fact, that we cannot be sure to achieve an adequately high radiation dose in residual tumor tissue with ^{131}I under these circumstances (Glanzmann, Horst 1979) and that we know, that even infiltrating neoplastic residues can effectively be controlled by teleradiotherapy for many years (Leisner et al. 1982). The technique should be based on the use of a telecobalt-irradiation or particle accelerator system and irradiated tissue volumes should be determined where possible with isodose lines on the basis of radiographs, CT-scanning and/or sonography (Harmer 1977). In general 2 fields are selected, sparing the cervical spine, larynx and trachea, frequently somewhat tilted towards the mediastinum. In these areas a focal dose of 60 Gy (e.g. 40 + 20, 2 Gy/day) should be applied in a period of up to 3 months (Tubiana et al. 1977). General and local side-effects can usually be controlled by administration of Vitamin-B-complex, methylprednisolone and locally effective agents such as viscose xylocaine etc. (Klein et al. 1976). In cases with large residual tumors the initial dose may be higher and local reactions such as edema of the laryngeal mucosa should be avoided by initially high doses of prednisolone-derivatives (Riccabona 1986). When there is a significant infiltration of the oesophagus it may be beneficial to place a gastric tube at the beginning of the radiotherapy course to avoid problems in nutrition. The irradiated skin areas should be protected by panthenol cream or similar preparations. Results of such teleradiotherapeutic methods compared with results of other treatment programs in relevant groups of patients are shown in Table 34. Late and sometimes severe complications were observed in the days of conventional x-ray therapy and inadequate dose calculations in the irradiated area (zum Winkel 1964). Radiodermatitis and radionecrosis in the neck and radionecrosis of

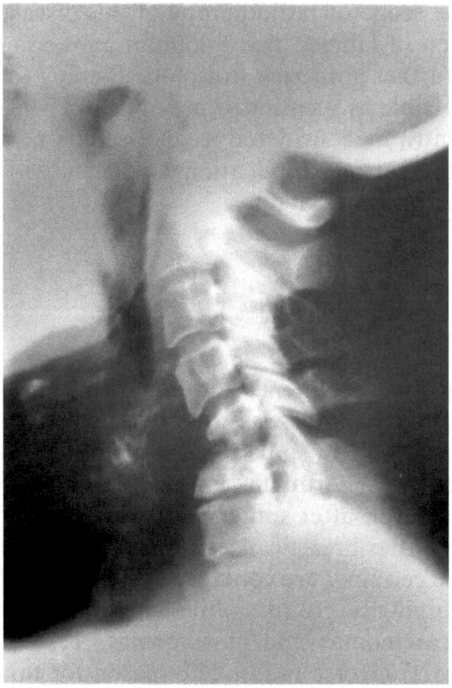

Fig. 41. Radionecrosis of C5/C4 after percutaneous conventional radiotherapy 10 years after unradical surgery for badly differentiated follicular Ca. Paraplegia, death. At autopsy no evidence of tumor

Table 34. Indications and results of percutanous radiotherapy of thyroid cancer

Indications	Results
1) Inoperable primary tumors without ^{131}I-uptake	Occasional positive effects
2) Local irradiation after surgery for undifferentiated or medullary carcinoma and sarcomas	Is always included in our therapeutic program (5 year survival rate 70%) possibly together with ^{131}I and/or chemotherapy
3) Local irradiation after palliative surgery of the primary lesion	
4) Local irradiation after surgery in patients of >45 years	
5) Local irradiation in patients with lymph node or mediastinal metastases	
6) Radiotherapy of metastases without ^{131}I-uptake (either solitary or with relevant symptoms)	Frequently adequate palliation over 3–18 months

cervical vertebrae (Fig. 41) have been reported and it was a terrible experience to see tumor-free patients suffer severely from such alterations:

Case P.A., female, 71.25.03.15

Near total thyroidectomy 1962 for follicular thyroid carcinoma (elsewhere). Postoperative conventional radiotherapy. In fall 1964 pain in left hip and thigh.

Radiograms of pelvis and thigh normal. On ^{131}I-scan suspect activity in pelvis. Therefore 80 mCi ^{131}I on March 12th, 1965. Patient then feeling better, definite uptake in pelvis on the left side in June 1965. 100 mCi ^{131}I on June 12th, 1965, even though pelvis radiograms were normal. In February 1966 increasing dyspnoea, chest films show suspect shadow in left lung. 90 mCi ^{131}I on February 2nd, 1966. In October 1966 induration of left parotid area, other findings normal. Parotidectomy in November 1966 (fibrosis of parotid gland with stenosis of parotid duct). Patient then doing well until February 1968: dysphagia, nausea, weight loss. Moderate diffuse infiltration on left side of neck (Scar? Tumor?). Then spontaneous improvement. Skin on neck shows radiodermatitis, patient is taking thyroid hormone. In March 1973 severe swallowing problems. No abnormal ^{131}I-uptake, chest film normal, barium swallow reveals fistula of oesophagus. Surgery shows severe scarring of tissue in neck (radionecrosis), gastrostomy and drainage performed, no evidence of tumor. October 1973: pains in neck, films show destruction of C5–7, no abnormal ^{131}I-uptake. Improvement with orthopedic support of cervical spine and doing well until 1976 when severe dysphagia is reported. Endoscopy shows recurrent severe stricture of the oesophagus, endoscopic dilatation, perforation, death from mediastinitis on June 16th, 1976. Post mortem: no evidence of tumor, severe fibrosis of neck and mediastinum, mediastinitis after endoscopic perforation of the oesophagus.

Today, however, we feel that radiotherapy planning has reached a level, where this adjunctive kind of treatment should be employed freely in thyroid cancer patients belonging to "high-risk-groups" (Kagan et al. 1974) and that it even can provide significant palliation in cases with large inoperable tumors for a period which can last for many months: case Z.H. (see page 56).

Necessity and modalities of such a treatment should always be discussed in detail with the patient, with surgeons and radiotherapists as well as nuclear medicine specialists.

Teleradiotherapy for Metastatic Thyroid Cancer

As in other malignancies teleradiotherapy can be valuable to control pain or tumor growth especially due to bone metastases (Riccabona 1980) when no radioiodine uptake exists in the relevant lesion. Considering the remarks made in the chapter on "surgery", however, one should not wait for weeks to see whether or not e.g. a spinal metastasis of thyroid cancer will respond to radiotherapy, while we waste precious time needed to save the patient from paraplegia or pathological fractures and when surgical interventions can also be considered. On the other hand focal doses of approx. 40 Gy can – in many instances – stabilize metastatic lesions for a long time (Halnan 1975) and provide help for the suffering patients. Radiation reactions due to simultaneous irradiation of the gastrointestinal tract or bladder are controlled by the same medication as mentioned for radiotherapy in the neck, sometimes adding spasmolytic preparations. Mediastinal metastases can also represent an interesting target for teleradiotherapy if no ^{131}I-uptake exists. Large, obstructing tumor masses can frequently be shrunk, so that the patients remain without congestion, breathing problems or dysphagia for a long time.

Finally it should be stated once again, that we should be aware of the important beneficial effects of teleradiotherapy in the management of thyroid cancer and that we should apply this sort of treatment whenever it seems appropriate but not on a routine basis in all thyroid cancer cases.

^{131}I-therapy

It is well known that even metastatic thyroid cancer can effectively be controlled by ^{131}I in large doses (Horst 1985). When this therapeutic approach was described decades ago, the medical community hoped that with such an approach all thyroid cancer cases could be cured. In the meantime we know better. Depending on variations in the distribution of thyroid cancer types only 40–75% of thyroid carcinomas will take up ^{131}I in amounts, from which therapeutic effects can be expected (Tubiana 1982). Furthermore a primary ^{131}I-uptake in the malignancy is a rather rare phenomenon (Spencer 1978) which we have seen in only 15% of our carcinoma cases. In the other patients radioiodine concentrations in thyroid cancer were observed only after surgical or radioiodine elimination of normal thyroid tissue. At present the value of general radioiodine treatment after surgery for thyroid carcinoma is a matter of sometimes vivid discussions (Snyder et al. 1983). In a similar manner as mentioned in the chapter on surgical therapy, some groups argue, that patients belonging to "low-risk-groups" (well differentiated tumor types, T_0-T_3, N_1, M_0, young age group) should not receive ^{131}I to eliminate thyroid remnants. Other authors and we ourselves propose, that in view of the uncertain long-time course of the disease, radioiodine ablation of thyroid remnants after surgery for thyroid carcinoma should be carried out routinely (Benua et al. 1982). For us only well encapsulated highly differentiated "microcarcinomas" ($\varnothing < 1.5$ cm) discovered by chance in patients below 40 years of age are spared from adjunctive ^{131}I-treatment. One reason for this aggressive strategy is the fact, that in many instances it is only after application of a large ablation dose that metastases become apparent in patients which should have been operated "radically":

Case W.F., male, 95.14.01.10

Thyroidectomies in 1924 and 1944. Since 1959 again recurrent nodular goiter on the right, euthyroid, neck and chestfilms regular. Proposed surgery refused by patient. In December 1976 patient was seen again, because of further growth of nodule in spite thyroid hormone therapy. Euthyroid, on scan nodule hot, thyroid lobes neither visualized on scan nor palpable. Chest film regular. Now removal of subcutaneous nodule on January 13th, 1977. Histology: Follicular carcinoma. On postoperative ^{131}I-scan now small thyroid lobes visible, also 2 foci with ^{131}I-uptake in chest. 150 mCi ^{131}I on January 28th, 1977, teleradiotherapy (60 Gy). Patient then doing well until February 1978. Palpable mass in left thyroid region, cytology: Pap. V, radiograms regular, BSR normal. Reintervention on March 7th, 1978. Near total thyroidectomy. Histology: follicular carcinoma. On postoperative scan no abnormal ^{131}I-uptake. In October 1982 no complaints, thyroglobulin 88 ng/ml (values in 1981 still normal), on chest film metastasis in right lung, withdrawal of hormone therapy, 144 mCi ^{131}I on January 12th, 1983. May 1985: Only small residues of lung metastases, thyroglobulin 37 ng/ml, ^{131}I-scan normal, patient doing well, except problems with hypertension and diabetes.

These abnormal radioiodine distribution patterns can frequently be observed also in patients with malignancies which theoretically should not show ^{131}I-concentrations in tumor tissue on the basis of histological reports (Riccabona 1981). It is certainly not adequate, however, to apply e.g. 30 mCi (= 1.1 GBq) to eliminate thyroid remnants after surgery on a routine basis (Snyder et al. 1983). Our aim must be:

a) to eliminate thyroid remnants with a dose of 500 Gy depending on uptake, size of remnants and effective half-life of ^{131}I in the thyroid,
b) to destroy – if possible – existing metastases of thyroid cancer with doses of 60 – 500 Gy, taking into account acceptable whole body radiation doses.

It does not therefore seem justified to treat patients with thyroid cancer with an uptake in the thyroid remnants of $<2\%$ after 24 hrs and with a 48 hr whole-body retention of less than 3%. Even if with large tracer doses metastases of thyroid carcinomas can be visualized on scans the therapeutic dose rate would remain inadequate under such circumstances. This is also an important argument for us to apply ^{131}I-treatment only, if – after a tracer dose of 1 – 2 mCi of ^{131}I (37 – 74 MBq) – tumor tissue is seen on 24 hr scans. When you need 100 mCi (= 3.7 GBq) of ^{131}I to detect tumor tissues with very sensitive gamma-camera systems, jou can forget about therapeutic effects of ^{131}I! Such data will contribute to diagnostic staging but not to therapeutic decisions. On the other hand ^{131}I-therapy under such circumstances seems justified in any case of thyroid carcinoma except in cases of an existing pregnancy. Radioiodine can today be applied by capsules or solution. Capsules have 2 advantages, namely simpler handling for the treating doctor with less risk of contamination and no problems with ^{131}I-resorption in oral mucosa. Patients with a tendency to vomit and other swallowing problems should receive their dose after antiemetic premedication and sometimes in liquid form via a gastric tube. Do not forget to place an in-dwelling catheter in the bladder in severely ill patients for 48 hrs to avoid possible contamination of bed-sheets etc. by radioactive urine! Only in rare cases will i.v. application of sterile ^{131}I be necessary. In cases with a high ^{131}I-uptake in thyroid tumor masses dose rates of up to 20 mr/hr at a 1 m distance were observed. It is mandatory therefore to monitor the incorporated activity regularly after large dose ^{131}I-therapy and – if necessary – to restrict the exposure time per day of hospital personnel during their activities in dealing with "hot" patients. Plastic covers over matresses can also help to avoid contamination of beds.

With regard to our therapeutic strategy with ^{131}I the essential data are presented in Table 35 (Riccabona 1986). The beneficial effects of an intensive use of ^{131}I for treatment of thyroid cancer are shown in Table 36, which gives data that correlate well with literature reports (Horst 1985). The effect of treatment of metastases with adequate ^{131}I-uptake can be spectacular (Fig. 42) and indeed

Table 35. Methods of ^{131}I-therapy of thyroid cancer

Mode of therapy	Indication	Methods	Therapeutic goal
1) Ablation of thyroid remnants	After radical or palliative surgery of thyroid carcinoma (no C-cell tumors!) regardless of age	If possible 50000 rads but < 100 mCi	"Athyroidism"
2) "Curative" ^{131}I-therapy of tumor residues or metastases	^{131}I-uptake in tumor residues or metastases regardless of age and histology	Single doses of 100–250 mCi in intervals of 3–4 months during 1 year	Elimination of tumor residues or metastases
3) "Palliative" ^{131}I-therapy	If 2) did not achieve therapeutic goal, ^{131}I-uptake in tumor residues or metastases persists and tumor shows progression. Regardless of age and histology	Single doses of 100–150 mCi over years (every 6th – 12th month) stay as long as possible below 1 Ci!	Palliation of symptoms, impairment of tumor growth over longest possible period

Note: No ^{131}I-therapy during pregnancy!

Table 36. Results of ^{131}I-therapy

With ^{131}I		Without ^{131}I
1 year survival	90%	88%
3 year survival	65%	60%
5 year survival	48%	20%
10 year survival	40%	–

Table 37. Complications after ^{131}I-therapy of thyroid cancer

Type of complication	Frequency	Prophylaxis and therapy
Radiation parotitis	Occasional	Chewing gum, lemon, sour drops
Radiation thyroiditis in thyroid remnants	Occasional	Prednisolone
Pulmonary fibrosis in diffuse lung metastases	Rare	Theophylline prednisolone
Leucemia	Rare (after total doses of > 1 Ci)	Chemotherapy
Aplastic anemia or panmyelopathy	Rare (after total doses of > 1 Ci)	Vit. B complex prednisolone transfusions (anabolic preparations)
Thyrotoxicosis	Rare	Antithyroid drugs prednisolone

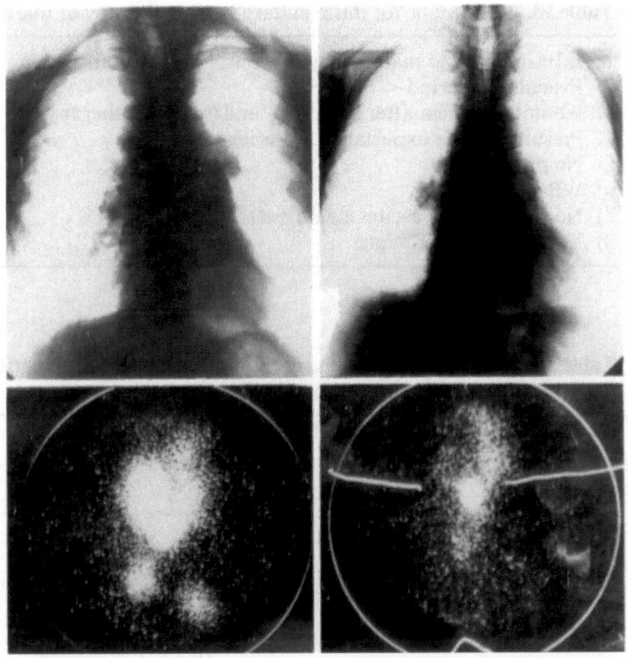

Fig. 42. Therapeutic effect of ^{131}I treatment of follicular thyroid Ca in 78 yr. old male patient.
Left: Above: mediastinal and lung metastases of thyroid Ca on chest film. *Below:* scan showing intense uptake in metastatic lesions.
Right: Above: after 250 mCi ^{131}I nearly normal chest film. *Below:* Poor uptake in thyroid region, mediastinum and lung. Patient died at age 85 of pneumonia

many patients with metastatic thyroid cancer can be cured by this sort of therapy (Pochin 1971). On the other hand complications due to radioiodine therapy are also known (Table 37) (Benua et al. 1962) but can be overcome usually. Overall ^{131}I-therapy of thyroid carcinoma can provide important possibilities even in cases with distant metastases of thyroid cancer if it is applied appropriately. It must be stressed, however, that the large required doses usually make the patient a "radiation source" for several days after therapy and that patients must therefore be admitted to specially equipped wards for a few days (Emrich 1979). Iodine exposure (contrast media etc!) prior to radioiodine therapy must be avoided to allow sufficient ^{131}I-uptake in thyroid cancer (see above). There is no evidence on the other hand that pregnancies starting 6 months after large-dose ^{131}I-treatment of thyroid cancer could suffer from genetic radiation effects (Rösler, Moser 1984) if the disease is under control and if the patient remains euthyroid with adequate thyroid hormone therapy.

Intracavitary Radioisotope Treatment

Pleural effusions due to carcinosis of the pleural cavity can occur in advanced stages of thyroid cancer (Riccabona 1979). Sometimes such syndromes can be controlled by ^{131}I-therapy but in other cases – without sufficient radioiodine uptake in pleural lesions – the intracavitary application of ^{90}Y-colloid can be appropriate (Siegel et al. 1956). This kind of therapy is performed in cases with rapidly refilling effusions in chest or abdomen (Table 38) but with an expected

Table 38. Indications for intracavitary isotope therapy of malignant effusions

1) Effusions due to malignancy in pleural cavity or abdomen
2) Evacuation period < 10 days
3) No improvement after hormone- and/or chemotherapy
4) Presumable life expectance > 3 weeks
5) No pregnancy
6) WBC > 3000
7) No subileus (for ascites treatment)
8) No effusions with septa

Table 39. Results of intracavitary therapy of pleural and peritoneal carcinosis in comparison to other intracavitary therapy programs

	Source	n	Side effects	Method	Objectively positive results	Duration of remission ($\bar{x}$)
Intracavitary cytostatic drugs	Fracchia et al.	138	43% (3.6% [a])	Cycloph. Thiotepa	27.5%	8.8 m.
	Weisberger et al.	88	?	Cycloph.	63.5%	?
	Mark et al.	32	47% (6.2% [a])	Mechlor-ethamine	?	?
	Anderson et al.	60	50% (13.2% [a])	Cycloph.	47.0%	3 m.
	Anderson, Brincker	86	41%	Thiotepa	37.0%	?
Intracavitary tetracycline	Zaloznik et al.	30	7.7%	Tetracycline + chest tube	69.0%	4.9 m.
Intracavitary radioactive colloids	Emrich	131	5%	^{198}Au-coll. ^{32}P-Cr-phosph.	38.8%	?
	Scheer et al.	239	?	^{198}Au-coll.	46.9%	?
	Own material	62	8.1%	^{90}Y-coll. (^{198}Au-coll.)	68.5%	4.5 m.

[a]) Severe side effects due to serious bone marrow damage

lifespan of more than 3 weeks. As about 10% of the given activity can be absorbed into the circulation a white blood cell count of at least 3000 WBC/mm^3 should be present (Riccabona 1986a). After withdrawal of the fluid 90–120 mCi (3.25–4.45 GBq) of ^{90}Y-colloid are administered in the afflicted cavity together with 40 mg of cristalline methylprednisolone in a volume of 50–150 ml NaCl. Patients should change position regularly during the first hours after therapy to permit a homogenous distribution of ^{90}Y all over the treated space. Effusions with septa should therefore be – if possible – excluded from such therapeutic programs or treated by separate applications of dose fractions in the different compartments of the exsudate under x-ray or scintillation scanning control after intracavitary application of radioactive gamma-emitting colloids (Vider et al. 1976). Overall it should be mentioned that in such clinical situations intracavitary radiocolloid therapy produces the same results with less morbidity than intracavitary treatment with cytostatic drugs (Riccabona 1984) or tetracycline (Zaloznik et al. 1983) (Table 39) and that satisfactory long-term remissions can be obtained frequently.

To finish this chapter on radionuclide therapy of thyroid cancer I would like to mention once more the future potential for treatment with ^{131}I-labeled thyroglobulin antibodies. Preliminary results are available but scarce and the technique may provide another important tool for the control of thyroid cancer.

3 Chemotherapy

Primarily cytostatic therapy of thyroid cancer was tried in desperate cases in which the full potential of surgery and radiation therapy had been exhausted (Riccabona 1976). Even with rather primitive combinations of cytostatic drugs, however, considerable remissions were be observed (Benker, Reinwein 1983) and therefore chemotherapy of malignant thyroid disease is today considered as a valuable alternative together with other therapy programs (Horst 1985). There are, however, significant differences in opinions concerning the clinical value of such medications. While some groups insist, that they should – also today – be given only in "desperate cases" (no other therapeutic approaches available in patients with tumor progression and relevant symptoms) (Benker et al. 1977), others argue, that in the age of sensitive tumor-marker-radioassays they should also be administered to patients with rising tumor-marker titers without clinical evidence of recurrent or metastatic disease (Durie 1981), as smaller tumor cell populations can certainly be more efficiently controlled than clinically detectable tumor masses. The well-known side effects of possibly aggressive chemotherapy programs together with the individually uncertain outcome (responders – non-responders!) make it difficult in some instances to convince patients who are doing well – e.g. with an elevated calcitonin- or thyroglobulin value – of the necessity for chemotherapy. Furthermore it is mentioned even in publications of recent origin, that thyroid cancer in general does not respond adequately to chemotherapy (Poster et al. 1981). Finally the choice, dosage and application schedule for all proposed cytostatic agents is still a matter of discussion (Samonigg et al. 1983). So – before starting chemotherapy of thyroid cancer – we must be aware of three facts:

a) we do not know which cytostatic drug(s) we should give
b) we do not know in which dose the agent(s) should be applied and
c) we do not know if the patient will respond positively to such a medication or if side-effects will finally outweigh possible benefits.

Such a situation would seem to rule out chemotherapy of thyroid cancer in general compared with other situations in clinical medicine. Yet, the literature does include reports on sometimes spectacular remissions of wide-spread thyroid malignancy achieved with a variety of chemotherapeutic programs and so any concerned doctor will have to consider such possible therapies especially in

Table 40. Chemotherapy of thyroid cancer (programs) cases with inoperable recurrences or metastases, no ^{131}I-therapy, no teleradiotherapy possible

	Agents applied	Therapy course
1)	6-Mercaptopurine Cyclophosphamide Procarbazine 5-Fluorocil Amethopterine Vinblastin (adjuvant therapy: Methylprednisolone Vit. B, C, Belladonna 19-Norandrostenolone)	Over 1 week p.o, i.m., i.v., Repeat every 4 weeks
2a) b) c)	D-oxo-rubicine (Adriamycin) Vinblastin or Vincristin (adjuvant therapy: e.g. Thiethylperazine Adriamycin total [a)] Dose < 500 mg)	a) 60 mg b) 0.1 mg/kg body weight c) 0.05 mg/kg body weight repeat every 4–6 weeks
3a) b) c)	Cis-platinum (Abiplatin) Vincristin Adriamycin [a)] total dose < 500 mg (adjuvant therapy: Thiethylperazine, fluid, mannose)	
4)	Aclacinomycine (typically 4 courses à 4 × 40 mg)	

[a)] = Doxorubicine

patients belonging to a prognostically fatal group with thyroid cancer, taking into account the fact that he is dealing with an unbalanced body of case material.

What can we do?

Suggested chemotherapeutic programs include many of the currently available cytostatic drugs (Table 40), without any evidence of the specificity of a particular agent (Alexeiva, Figusch et al. 1978). Some dosage programs are attached to Table 40 (Riccabona 1986).

When should we do it?

In view of the uncertain beneficial effects of any of the mentioned chemotherapeutic programs we would certainly not suggest applying them as "adjunctive chemotherapy" even in cases with undifferentiated carcinoma or medullary carcinoma without evidence of tumor residues or metastases after surgery. The only exception to this rule might be "malignant lymphoma" of the thyroid (Horst 1985), but in our limited experience of this disease ($n = 6$) it was always possible to control it by adequate surgery and local radiotherapy.

A clear decision can be made in cases where there is no response to other forms of treatment, tumor progression and relevant symptoms. For these patients chemotherapy remains the only chance they have and one should try any of the different programs freely, if the general condition of the patient permits such an aggressive strategy (Harada et al. 1981). In this context the radiosensitizing properties of several chemotherapeutic agents should also be mentioned, which might overall improve the prognosis of thyroid cancer patients in some cases. The most difficult group of patients to handle by applying cytostatic drug is probably the one made up of cases – as mentioned above – with rising tumor marker levels, no clinical evidence of tumor growth and no other therapeutic possibilities available (Hellman et al. 1980). At present we are trying a rather "harmless" chemotherapy program (Samonigg et al. 1983) on several such patients, but we cannot give any long-term results at present.

What can we expect from it?

Of course we can distinguish between responders and non-responders. Whatever the cytostatic drug program, we can in general assume an incidence of approx. 30–49% of responders (Horst 1985). Data are so far inadequate to determine which types of thyroid cancers respond to certain chemotherapeutic agents and which show no positive effect of cytostatic therapy. Overall, however, the benefits of chemotherapy applied under the conditions as mentioned previously are significant (Oberdisse et al. 1980) (Table 41) in terms of life-span and palliation effects:

Case G.A., female, 30.02.08.14

Spontaneous recurrent nerve paralysis on the left in summer 1968 with hoarseness and growth of nodular goiter. September 1968: Lobectomy on the left, resection on the right. Histology: "Proliferating adenoma", without definite criteria for malignancy. In view of the clinical situation radiotherapy after surgery (40 Gy). August 1970: Neck regular, mass in right mediastinum, no ^{131}I-uptake. Nevertheless 100 mCi ^{131}I in November 1970. Telecurietherapy on thoracic lesion (30 Gy). March 1971: Patient feeling well, tumor mass in mediastinum somewhat larger, ^{131}I-uptake present: 120 mCi of ^{131}I. March 1973: Pulmonary metastases, hilar mass unchanged, local lymph nodes on the left neck side. Removal of lymph nodes on March 28th, 1973 (histology: Metastases of papillary

Table 41. Results and complications of chemotherapy

Results	Complications	
45% 3 yr. survival vs.	Leukopenia	20%
3% 3 yr. survival in similar group without chemotherapy	Panmyelopathy	0.5%
15% 5 yr. survival vs.	Vomiting	70%
0% survival without chemotherapy	Alopecia	~50%
4% 10 yr. survival.	(Not yet with Aclacinomycine)	

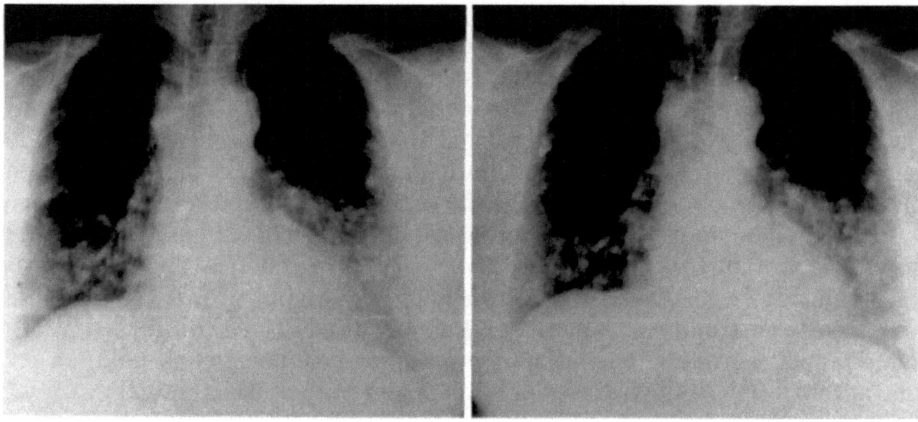

Fig. 43. Example of effect of chemotherapy. 10 years after initial therapy of follicular thyroid Ca 63 year old female patient had developed mediastinal and lung metastases. No ^{131}I-uptake (*left*). Control chest film 2 years later shows no progression of disease (*right*)

carcinoma), teleradiotherapy (30 Gy). June 1973: Lung metastases larger, polychemotherapy started as no ^{131}I-uptake was present. Remission (after Adriamycin and Vincristin) until November 1976, then local recurrence in the neck, thoracic lesions with slight progression, patient still doing well (Fig. 43). February 1977: removal of local recurrences, next series of chemotherapy started. April 1978: Increasing dyspnoea, coughing, progression of thoracic metastases, weight loss, weakness. Death on January 22nd, 1979 due to "cardiac failure" with increasing signs of progressive neoplastic disease.

Complications from chemotherapy are well known in general (Riccabona et al. 1976) and they exist in the same pattern also in cases with thyroid cancer. We so far have never lost a patient due to chemotherapy and other symptoms or complications are – given appropriate treatment – usually transient and can be controlled (Benker et al. 1984). It must be mentioned, that some potent cytostatic preparations show a cumulative toxicity especially concerning myocardial function and kidney function (Vogl et al. 1976). The recommended total dose limits (e.g. 500 mg Doxorubicin/m^2 body surface, 70 mg Cisplatin chloride/m^2 body surface) should therefore be respected and for any new course of chemotherapy cardiac function (ECG, radionuclide ventriculography with gated bloodpool technique) (Lenzhofer et al. 1983) as well as renal function (radionuclide clearance of ^{99m}Tc-DTPA and radioiodine-hippurate, endogenous creatinine clearance, BUN, creatinine, urinalysis) should be checked together with blood counts and liver function tests. With these precautions important therapeutic effects can frequently be obtained with chemotherapy. One problem, however, is the patient's compliance to such treatments. Even as hair-loss is transient and can be reduced by the use of cooling caps on the head during administration of the preparations, some patients are so worried by this phenomenon together with nausea and vomiting that they refuse further chemotherapy. When talking about "failures" concerning the therapeutic effect of cytostatic drugs one should not only consider the "non-responders" but also the considerable number of patients – who even after adequate information about their disease state and remaining therapeutic possibilities – refuse further chemotherapy after perhaps one or two courses.

What can we do in the future?

In research programs on thyroid cancer (EORTC) the specific effects of various cytostatic drugs on malignancies of the thyroid gland should be studied carefully (Benker, Reinwein 1983). From a human point of view such "blind" or "double-blind" studies are difficult to perform, as doctors, who are convinced that chemotherapy could help their severely ill patients, will not be ready to administer only a placebo-preparation. Furthermore continuing research on cytostatic therapy is increasing the number of available substances year by year. One suggestion would be therefore to collect data on clinical success in a multicenter study covering a whole continent in which – for a period of approx. 2 years – a participating center will use one single drug or a well defined combination of drugs in a given dosage in thyroid cancer patients eligible for such treatment programs. Thus, no physician must feel that "he is doing nothing" for the patient, the remission rates as well as the complications of different chemotherapeutic approaches will become apparent. On the other hand "placebo"-medication could be avoided because we know, what patients can expect for their life-span etc. without chemotherapy of classified thyroid cancers according to internationally accepted histological criteria and TNM-stages. Let us hope therefore that the cytostatic drugs now available can be tested carefully during the next few years, so that we will know, which drugs or drug combinations should be applied for the treatment of different types of thyroid cancer.

Together with the new possibilities of radioimmunotherapy cytostatic drugs might provide the most important progress in the management of wide-spread thyroid cancer in the future.

4 Thyroid Hormone Therapy

For decades the beneficial effects of thyroid hormone medication in large doses were noticed (Crile 1955) in the treatment of thyroid cancer patients. The reason for these effects seem to be a maximum suppression of pituitary TSH-secretion (Hüfner et al. 1975) as it was reported that TSH can promote also the growth of thyroid carcinoma (see previously). Whereas in the past desiccated thyroid was given for this purpose (100–500 mg/day!) (Hoffmann 1977), synthetic preparations of l-thyroxine, l-triiodothyronine or combinations of both hormones are currently in use (Pickardt 1984). Table 42 shows different doses recommended by several groups. At this point it seems appropriate to mention also possible side-effects of such large thyroid hormone doses on the nervous system and the cardiovascular system (De Groot, Stanbury 1975): Some

Table 42. Daily thyroid hormone doses in management of thyroid-cancer (doses for adults 1.73 m² body-surface)

	Desiccated thyroid	I-T4	I-T3	T4+T3 combinations (4:1 or 5:1)
"Suppressive" thyroid hormone therapy	~240 mg	150–200 mcg	~ 100 mcg	~150 mcg T4 +~50 mcg T3
Thyroid hormone substitution	~120 mg	100 mcg–150	~75 mcg	100 mcg T4 +25 mcg T3

authors suggest that patients after surgery and initial radiotherapy for thyroid carcinoma should be kept in a clinically tolerable state of "thyrotoxicosis factitia" (Thomas 1958), while other groups find that even with lower thyroid hormone doses TSH-secretion can be suppressed and side-effects can be avoided (especially in older patients with cardiac problems) (Clark 1981). Some centers prefer the rapidly available and rapidly metabolized triiodothyronine (Seissl et al. 1977), other the initially mild metabolic effects of pure thyroxine (Lamberg et al. 1977). Anyway we are convinced that TSH-receptor-assays in thyroid cancer tissue (see previously) could modify the therapeutic application of thyroid hormone significantly: It is useless – e.g. – to push a patient with well determined medullary carcinoma or with malignant hemangioendothelioma to the border of clinical "thyrotoxicosis factitia" with a high thyroid hormone dosage, such cases should be kept euthyroid after surgery with appropriate amounts of thyroid hormone but should not be subjected to "suppressive thyroid hormone therapy" (Horst 1985). On the other hand "suppressive doses" of thyroid hormone can be valuable (Balme 1954) in patients with well-differentiated thyroid adenocarcinomas (probably with positive TSH-receptor values in the tumor tissue).

Substitution of lacking thyroid hormone after initial therapy of thyroid cancer by appropriate medication is one thing, suppressive thyroid hormone treatment after primary therapy another, but – of course – thyroid hormone per se cannot cure thyroid malignancies.

There has also been some discussion about the superior value of triiodothyronine (T_3) in thyroid hormone therapy versus thyroxine (T_4) (Pickardt 1984). The arguments put forward for such an approach are, that T_3 inhibits TSH-secretion more effectively than T_4, that it is resorbed almost completely in the gastrointestinal tract and that – as it is metabolized rapidly (Oberdisse et al. 1980) – suppressive effects on radioiodine uptake studies will vanish in approx. 2 weeks after the medication is withdrawn. On the other hand the rapid and thorough resorption of an oral T_3-dose, which then binds to transport protein less than T_4 and is not subjected to conversion mechanisms (De Groot, Stanbury 1975) can produce unphysiological thyroid hormone spikes in tissue leading to cardiovascular and nervous side effects especially in elderly patients (Wenzel, Meinhold 1974). Desiccated thyroid on the other hand – which was the first drug used for hormone therapy of thyroid cancer and is still available in many countries – should (if possible) be avoided as it contains, of course, not only T_3 and T_4 but relatively large amounts of iodine in various molecules (De Groot, Stanbury 1975). The iodine load of a patient with thyroid carcinoma, however, can be critical if – as mentioned previously – radioiodine treatment seems essential. Basically we know that we can indeed substitute thyroid hormone output and even suppress TSH-secretion with all sorts of thyroid hormone preparations (Oberdisse et al. 1980). The choice of the prescribed drug in the individual case will therefore depend more on local availability, patient compliance (e.g. T_3-preparations should be taken 2–4 times per day!) and the clinical situation: In cases in which repeated ^{131}I-treatments are likely over a period of less than a year, T_3-preparations could be preferred as patients can be kept euthyroid over most of the time between each therapy (Horst 1985) because T_3 must be stopped only 2–3 weeks before the next radioiodine application. If T_3 in adequate doses is not tolerated well by the patient, if it is not available or (see above) if patient compliance with this therapy is poor it is certainly possible to give such patients T_4 or T_3/T_4 combinations. The longer biological half-life of T_4 requires, however, that the medication be stopped 4–6 weeks before further ^{131}I-therapy (see previously) and if only desiccated thyroid can be prescribed such drugs must be withdrawn – when given in "suppressive" doses – 6–8 weeks before ^{131}I-therapy. In this context it should be mentioned, that for unknown reasons the dose levels used for suppressive thyroid hormone therapy vary considerably (Hoffmann et al. 1977): While some groups need 200–500 mcg of T_4/day (!) to obtain an adequate effect (Busnardo et al. 1981) others report similar results on TSH-suppression with doses of 100–200 mcg T_4/day (Svyatuklina et al. 1969). The same observations were made with other thyroid hormone preparations. This discrepancy can be explained either by variations in pharmacological stability of different thyroid hormone drugs or by different metabolic activity – especially of T_4 – in different populations (conversion-rates, hormone-receptor interaction etc.). It does not therefore seem justified to go ahead – e.g. – with 300 mcg of T_4/day for hormone therapy in thyroid cancer, but one should rather determine individual hormone dose levels on the basis of ultrasensitive TSH-radioassays or TRH-Tests taking into account also side-effects and patient compliance to achieve satisfactory results.

5 General Therapeutic Strategy

As mentioned several times in previous chapters thyroid cancer is certainly not "one" pathological entity but consists of a variety of really different diseases. It certainly is therefore very difficult to propose a general approach for therapy. However, in view of the chaotic proposals for the treatment of cancer sometimes made today – and not only for thyroid malignancies – the author is nevertheless convinced that some general guidelines for the management of thyroid cancer should be proposed. Just recently I heard of a colleague, who had said, that he had never seen a patient dying from papillary thyroid carcinoma and of another who told relatives of a patient with follicular carcinoma that any thera-

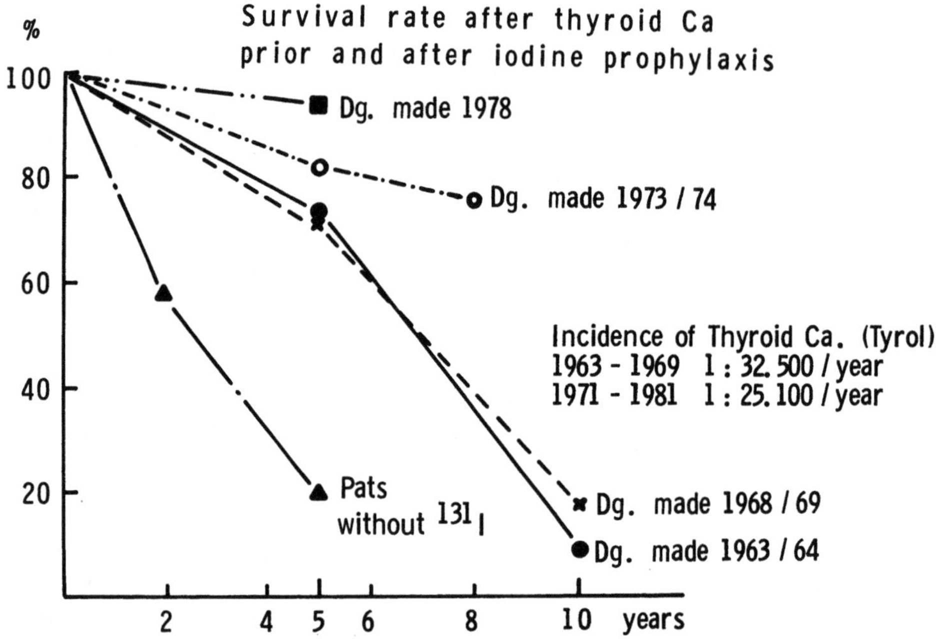

Fig. 44. Therapeutic results in thyroid Ca overall in own material over the past decades. Note significant improvement after ^{131}I-prophylaxis of endemic goiter became effective

peutic efforts would be useless. Between these two extreme positions an enormous variety of different attitudes exists, concerning the handling of patients with assorted forms and stages of thyroid malignancies (Horst 1985). All I can do under these circumstances according to my medical conscience is to present a model for the management of thyroid cancer with which during all the past years we have achieved considerable success with little side-effects in our approx. 1500 patients (Fig. 44). There certainly should be no therapeutic over-kill but even less should there be therapeutic resignation or negligence when we are confronted with thyroid cancer. In view of the biological pecularities of this disease it is extremely important for satisfactory long-term results not to lose interest in the patient once "appropriate" therapy has been administered but to follow-up the patients for many years and even decades (Riccabona 1986). A 5-year-survival in thyroid cancer is certainly no proof of a real cure!

Follow-up Programs in Thyroid Cancer

Any follow-up program after thyroid cancer will have to start with the decision about what to tell the patient and his family concerning the nature, spread and prognosis of the disease. If patients are discharged believing that they had only simple goiter, they frequently tend to neglect prescribed medication and adequate follow-up appointments. If on the other hand a patient – e.g. at an age of 55 years with metastatic poorly differentiated follicular carcinoma and with lesions in lungs and bone – is informed precisely about the chances for a long-term cure even with all the available therapeutic facilities some will have a nervous break-down (going as far a suicide!) or refuse any further treatment, because he or she may feel that all is lost. Several such patients then seek advice from obscure "cancer centers", see the local "Njanja" (= witch doctor) in developing countries, thus losing any chance for a cure or at least middle-term stabilization of their ailment. Between these 2 extremes there is a large variety of individual situations depending on the intellectual capacity of the patients, cooperation from his family and local physicians, pathology, tumor stage and the willingness of the afflicted person to fight for life. Under such circumstances it is impossible of course to "prescribe" general guidelines for adequate patient information, which – on the other hand – is a significant factor for the implementation of appropriate follow-up programs. It takes a lot of psychological knowledge and experience as well as a close relationship with the patient to be able – at least in most cases – to inform the patient in the right way, to convince his family of the necessity and benefits of a long-term follow-up and to establish a proper, sincere and active relationship between patient and treating doctor. This fact has been known for more than 2000 years (Ebers 1875), has sometimes been forgotten in the last century but is increasingly accepted again today (Illich 1976). Ultimately therefore the final success of therapy for thyroid cancer will depend not only on the ability and technical finesse of the treating doctors but also on the active cooperation of the patients.

Before presenting several types of follow-up programs in detail I would like to stress a few points, which in my personal experience and opinion, seem essential for the efficacity of long-term treatment and repeated check-ups:

a) Tell the patient that he did not have a simple goiter but that there was at least a tendency to malignancy,
b) Tell the patient that thyroid cancer in comparison with many other malignant lesions can be controlled effectively in the majority of cases if the prescribed medication is taken and long-term follow-up is carried out meticulously,

c) Tell the patient that he can always call or come if something worries him or if he has pain, breathing problems etc.
d) If you plan ^{131}I-therapy inform female patients that they should not become pregnant for 6 months after therapy and advise them on ways of avoiding pregnancies.
e) Inform patients due for ^{131}I-therapy, chemotherapy and radiotherapy about possible side-effects. In good conscience you can tell them that such symptoms are usually transitory and can – in the long run – effectively be controlled.
f) Give patients with wide-spread disease, which you have perhaps treated for many years and in which all the therapeutic possibilities are exhausted another follow-up appointment in several months. If you do not, they will feel let down by you and abandoned, which would mean a severe emotional trauma for such severely ill patients.

Regional differences in the attitude of a given population to malignant disease in general should certainly be respected and – as mentioned above – one should seek the informated cooperation of the patient's family and other committed friends. For many people the diagnosis "cancer" still means a verdict of death after a period of terrible suffering. We know, that this is not true for most cases with thyroid malignancy. We should therefore make every effort to break this prejudice against cancer in general and thyroid cancer especially, because we can then probably convince the public in 1–2 decades that most thyroid cancer patients can indeed be cured. Resignation on the part of patients on religious grounds can sometimes be overcome with arguments, that the patient does not know "god's will" or his "karma" and has to act according to his religious convictions as long as it is physically and mentally possible.

We mentioned the important effects of adequate thyroid hormone medication. Today it is important in some countries to inform patients that these thyroid hormone tablets are not "toxic drugs", no "dangerous chemical preparations", but that they are their own bodies' hormone which substitutes for the organism what his removed thyroid cannot provide any more. One could probably go on for many pages describing all the problems which must be handled by therapists of patients with thyroid cancer to achieve adequate patient compliance with treatment and follow-up. In the last resort, however, it will remain a success-story of genuine human cooperation if such programs can be carried out well.

Overall I am aware of the fact that these last few lines have little to do with "medical science", there are few statistics (Table 43), no formulae, no well-documented procedures. I nevertheless felt, that it was necessary to mention also the problems of psychological management of thyroid cancer patients in a book dealing with this disease and the comments should rather be considered as part of the age-old "ars medici" which was so important for ancient physicians and which we should not forget today.

After these general remarks well-defined follow-up programs will be proposed. They are tailored to the specific problems and therapeutic approaches of several types of thyroid cancer. With all the above-mentioned problems of

Table 43. Follow-up system after thyroid Ca

6 weeks after ^{131}I-therapy (program 1) Clinical exam, FT_4, TRH, TG, calcium, BC, ENT	Therapy ← ↓ Program 1 ↓ Program 2
3–4 months after ^{131}I-therapy (program 2) Thyroid hormone off for 4 weeks, ^{131}I-whole-body scan (1.0–2.0 mCi), TSH, TG, BC, chest film, ENT (calcium)	↓ Program 3 ↓
6–9 months after ^{131}I-therapy (program 3) Clinical exam, FT_4, TRH, TG, BC, bone scan, chest film	Program 4 ↓ Program 3 after 18 months ↓
12 months after ^{131}I-therapy (program 4) clinical exam, FT_4, TRH, TG, BC, chest film (perhaps also after T_4-withdrawal ^{131}I-whole-body-scan as above)	Program 4 after 24 months ↓ Regular follow-up every 6–12 months (program 3 or 4)

histological and pathophysiological classifications of thyroid malignancies it nevertheless seems appropriate for practical purposes to consider the 4 different programs for follow-up, presented on the next pages.

"Follow-up" denotes the complex of those diagnostic procedures required after initial therapy of the primary disease which enable the therapist without regard of primarily "radical" or "unradical" treatment of thyroid cancer to select adequate treatment for metastases or recurrences in due time. It also includes measures to monitor the metabolic situation and adjust it to an optimal situation and to treat complications of previous therapy.

1 Follow-up after Differentiated Thyroid Carcinoma

Programs depend more on clinical stage than on histology. Papillary and follicular carcinomas as well as "Hürthle-cell-tumors" are – for practical reasons – managed in the same way (Heinze 1984). Another important factor for the decision as to which follow-up program should be chosen is the age of the patient, as thyroid carcinomas are clearly more aggressive above about 45 years of age than below that age (Dole 1969). After several modifications of more rigid and more loose concepts we adopted the program shown in Table 44 about 10 years ago (Riccabona, Unterkircher 1981). It recognizes the fact that thyroglobulin in serum as measured by RIA is a valuable tumor marker for differentiated carcinoma but it does not substitute whole body radioiodine uptake studies by this method in general (see previously). It emphasizes the necessity to check the hormonal situation of the patient at regular intervals and especially clinical and also radiological aspects during long-term follow-up. It leaves enough possibilities to adjust the follow-up program to individual clinical situations. It must be stressed once more that after differentiated thyroid carcinoma

Table 44. Follow-up of patients with differentiated thyroid adeno-Ca.

1st)	After surgery, ^{131}I-therapy (evtl. also radiotherapy), thyroid hormone, no iodine exposure.
2nd)	During the first 3 yrs. postop. follow-up 3×/year alternating with thyroid hormone medication (clinical exam, control of hormonal suppression, radiographs, blood count, TG, ESR) or after 4 weeks of thyroid hormone (^{131}I-studies, TG, T4, TSH, blood count, ESR, radiographs).
3rd)	After 3–5 yrs. program as in 2) but only 2×/yr.
4th)	After 5 yrs program as in 2) but only 1×/yr., after 10 yrs. program as in 2) but only every other year.
5th)	If ^{131}I-uptake in metastases, follow-up exams and possibly ^{131}I-therapy after 4 weeks off thyroid hormone until tumor remission is achieved or therapeutic possibilities are exhausted.
6th)	Adapt programs to clinical course!

follow-up intervals in apparently tumor free patients can be gradually extended to 1 and 2 years, but that follow-up studies should run for decades before a patient is finally discharged as "cured" (Tubiana 1982):

Case H.N., male, 34.07.01.35

Thyroidectomy (elsewhere) in 1952. Histology: Follicular (?) carcinoma. Lymph-node metastases in 1960 on the right, removal elsewhere. Since 1969 growth of recurrent goiter, patient did not take any medication. On first admission (Feburary 15th, 1971) firm recurrent nodular goiter on the right, suspect lymph nodes on right side of the neck. On thyroid scan ^{131}I-uptake in recurrence and in lymph nodes. Chest films regular, recurrent nerve paralysis on the left. Near total thyroidectomy on February 19th, 1971 with modified neck dissection. Histology: Follicular carcinoma. 120 mCi ^{131}I on March 4th, 1971. Teleradiotherapy (50 Gy). In fall 1971 palpable lymph-nodes on right side of neck with ^{131}I-uptake, chest films normal. Radical neck dissection on October 12th, 1971, 120 mCi ^{131}I on February 2nd, 1972. Since then patient doing well, ^{131}I-scans, chest films and thyroglobulin normal. Euthyroid under thyroid hormone medication.

If at such a check-up even after years metastases or recurrences of the original tumor are detected, appropriate treatment should be administered as mentioned in the relevant chapters and follow-up intervals must go back to the original schedule. Patients – at least in central Europe – initially accept the follow-up studies mostly knowing that they had or have cancer. When many years have gone by, however, they tend to become negligent concerning follow-ups and medication with the result that they may end up in severe myxedematous states in some remote hospital (Forester 1963):

Case P.E., male, 71.13.03.22

Thyroidectomy for follicular Ca. in 1949 (elsewhere). Since spring 1977 swelling in left mandibular area, pain in left ear and left occipital region, dyspnoea, some weight loss. Removal of "necrotic bone" from acustic meatus in summer 1977. Never took thyroid medication, multiple "rheumatic" pains in skeleton. Hypothyroid patient, no evidence of tumor necrosis in the neck, multiple foci with ^{131}I-uptake in skull (parietal-temporal region on the left), lumbar spine, chest and pelvis. Radiograms of chest, spine and pelvis regular, irregular structures in left temporal region of the skull. 200 mCi ^{131}I on December 2nd, 1977. In the following years repeated difficulties in keeping patient on thyroid hormone. Usually he arrives in a severe myxedematous state and complains about nothing, does not keep check-up appointments. Definite tumor progression found in early summer 1978. 2×150 mCi ^{131}I, patient stays on ward until he is clearly euthyroid, is then instructed again about importance of regular check-ups and adequate thyroid hormone medication. Since then cooperative, several more ^{131}I-doses, still alive and doing quite well in 1985, euthyroid with thyroid hormone, tumor now constant, thyroglobulin 66 ng/ml.

It is therefore essential that local physicians and the patient's family are also informed about the necessity of proper medication and controls. Some people argue nowadays that regular radiological exams and large-dose radioiodine studies represent a dangerous radiation exposure with all the inherent risks (Stieve 1976). At a whole-body dose of approx. 100 mrad/year due to ^{131}I-studies, a dose of about 1000 mrad/year to the chest by routine x-ray exams and possibly a dose of approx. 300 mrad/year after bone scans with ^{99m}Tc-phosphate complexes, the dose increment is minimal and remains below the permitted radiation doses for professionally active personal in Radiology or Nuclear Medicine in most cases (Kaul, Roedler 1977). Some people also argue that the cost-benefit ratio of such follow-up programs would be out of proportion (Riccabona 1978). We know, however, what a severely ill, hospitalized thyroid cancer patient can cost per day and the financial burden of prolonged invalidity due to metastatic and slowly growing thyroid carcinoma (Table 45). Besides the humanitarian benefits of appropriate treatment at the appropriate time which is often only possible due to careful follow-up studies we are therefore convinced that such programs do not harm the patient and that they are actually cost-saving in many ways. Another problem remains: As mentioned earlier, differentiated thyroid carcinoma can – after many years – become a completely undifferentiated cancer (Orvoine et al 1983). This possibility must be born in mind at check-up exams and if it occurs further treatment and further follow-up must be of course adjusted to the changing situation. Such patients should then be handled as any anaplastic thyroid tumor.

Table 45. Economical aspects of management of thyroid cancer[a]

	"Therapeutic nihilism"	"active therapy"[b]
Mean survival	~20 months	10 years
Cost[c]	~36000 DM	~33000 DM

[a] Data according to austrian socio-economic situation, insurance policy and hospital costs
[b] "Active therapy": thyroidectomy, 2 telecobaltseries (60 Gy), ~500 mCi ^{131}I (mean value), hormonal substitution, 300 mg Doxorubicin and 30 mg Vincristin (mean value) over 5 years
[c] Cost: including sickness allowance for 2 person-household, costs of therapy and follow-up exams, pension for partner after death. Other socio-economic losses not considered!

2 Follow-up of Anaplastic Thyroid Cancer

For practical purposes again several types of thyroid cancer are included in this group. They are either anaplastic carcinomas of different patterns, sarcomas (with the exception of malignant lymphoma – see later) and hemangioendotheliomas without uptake of radioiodine in neoplastic tissue (see previously). This prognostically very poor group needs nevertheless our help as it can be provided. In view of some remarkable effects of chemotherapy and/or radiotherapy we never "write-off" a patient in whom such a diagnosis is made:

Case B.F., female, 10.02.02.14

Rapid growth of goiter since November 1971, tenderness of the tumor, dyspnoea, feeling tired. Admission on March 22nd, 1972: Patient euthyroid, firm large nodular goiter on the right *with* palpable lymph-nodes. Nodule cold, cytology Pap. V, chest films regular, moderate tracheal compression. Near total thyroidectomy on April 11th, 1972 with modified neck-dissection on the right. Histology: Fibrosarcoma of the thyroid. Teleradiotherapy (60 Gy), chemotherapy with Vincristin and Cyclophosphamide for 6 cycles. Postoperative ^{131}I-scans regular. Patient then doing well. In spring 1974: ^{67}Ga-scan: Suspect activity in right chest, also chest films suspect in this area. BSR 15/35. In fall 1974 definite evidence of solitary lung metastasis which was removed in September 1974. Next course of chemotherapy with Adriamycin and Vinblastin as radical removal of lung focus seemed doubtful. Patient euthyroid with thyroid hormone medication. In April 1975 recurrent lung metastases. Teleradiotherapy with 60 Gy. Chemotherapy continued. In the following months increasing dyspnoea, weight loss, anorexia. Chest films show large pleural effusion in right chest, lung metastases constant. Withdrawal of pleural fluid. Cytology Pap. V. Therefore intracavitary therapy with 76 mCi ^{90}Y-colloid on July 17th, 1975. Then general state gradually declining, no recurrent pleural effusion but progression of lung metastases. Further chemotherapy, death on March 15th, 1976.

Even if we can obtain a survival of only several years with the patient in a relatively good condition this may be crucial for many socio-economic reasons in a family, in a business etc. Knowing about the specific problems of this patient group we proposed (Riccabona 1986) a follow-up program as shown in Table 46. We also include in this group patients with metastatic lesions in the

Table 46. Follow-up after anaplastic thyroid carcinoma

1) After surgery, teleradiotherapy ^{131}I-ablation of thyroid remnants. Thyroid hormone (e.g. ~150 µg T_4/d), no iodine exposure.
2) After 3 months and 4 weeks off thyroid hormone TG, TSH, CEA, chest film, ^{131}I-whole body scan and if abnormal uptake, ^{131}I-therapy.
3) If no evidence of recurrence or metastases during 3 years follow-up exams 3×/year (physical, ESR, BC, FT_4, TSH, TG, chest film).
4) From 3–5 years as in 3) but only 2×/year.
5) After 5 years same as in 3) 1×/year.
6) In case of progression without ^{131}I-uptake chemotherapy.

thyroid of other malignant tumors because even then the effort is sometimes not wasted concerning the definite outcome:

Case J.H., male, 42.15.69.14

1960 right nephrectomy for hypernephroid Ca., subtotal thyroidectomy 1945. Since early 1968 rapid growth of nodular recurrent goiter. BSR 80/120. BC and urinalysis normal, chest film regular, on thyroid scan large, firm, cold nodule on the left. Cytology: Pap. IV. Near total thyroidectomy on October 10th, 1971. Histology "clear cell carcinoma" (later corrected: Metastasis of hypernephroid Ca.). Postoperative telecurietherapy (60 Gy), and 100 mCi of ^{131}I. Since then doing well, no evidence of metastases or recurrences clinically, on bone-scans or radiographs.

Our experience is, that even severely afflicted patients cooperate in such programs, often with significant medical, personal and socio-economic benefits as long as their doctors remain committed.

3 Follow-up of Medullary Carcinoma

The first step of any "follow-up-program" once the diagnosis has been firmly established should be – whenever possible – a family screening in which thyroid nodules, serum calcitonin (perhaps after alcohol-stimulation or pentagastrin-stimulation) should be registered (Williams 1981). Pathological findings in direct relatives of the patient should initiate a thorough examination of these individuals for manifestations of an MEN-syndrome (see previously) and ultimately provide adequate informations for therapeutic approaches (Baylin 1974). It is also important for the patient's prognosis, to know, whether he belongs to the group of medullary carcinoma in the framework of hereditary MEN-syndromes or not, as it has been reported that familiar medullary carcinoma has – in general – a poorer prognosis than sporadic cases (Williams 1979). Concerning the observations made in earlier chapters we would advise to check at least once after initial treatment ^{131}I-uptake patterns after thyroid hormone withdrawal just as in differentiated thyroid carcinomas (Riccabona 1984). For the rest, besides clinical exam, radiological check-ups and ultrasound studies, calcitonin and CEA-measurements will be the most essential parameters in the follow-up-programs as shown in Table 47 (Heinze 1984). We will see in the near future whether isotope scanning, with modified ^{99m}Tc-DMSA (Dimercaptosuccinate) radioiodinated MBG and ^{131}I-labeled CEA-antibodies (Horst 1985) will also play a significant role in such studies. Parameters defining an adequate thyroid hormone substitution must, of course, be included in check-up-studies (see above), but we will never need high dose suppressive thyroid hormone medication as only adequate substitution doses to maintain the patient in an euthyroid state are required. As shown above, diagnostic parameters for other manifestations (e.g. adrenals, intestine etc.) of MEN-syndromes should be obtained also in patients, in whom a suggestion of such a disease is present. Again it must be stressed, that follow-up programs should cover

Table 47. Follow-up of patients with medullary carcinomas

1st)	After surgery, irradiation and evtl. ^{131}I-therapy thyroid hormone, no iodine exposure as long as ^{131}I-uptake in residual tumor was not excluded. TCT, if positive, family screening.
2nd)	During 3 yrs. follow-up exams 3×/yr. under thyroid hormone medication (if ^{131}I-uptake was shown then as with diff. adeno-Ca.); including CEA, TCT, other programs as in Table 43
3rd)	From 3–5 yrs. program as in 2) 2×/yr.
4th)	After 5 yrs. program as in 2) 1×/yr., after 10 yrs. program as in 2) every other year.
5th)	In case of tumor progression chemotherapy (radiotherapy).
6th)	Adapt programs to clinical course!

decades if possible (Tubiana 1982), as late recurrences or metastases of medullary carcinoma are known. The problem of what to do with patients with elevated calcitonin and/or CEA-values and no other evidence of tumor progression has been discussed previously. Anyway such follow-up schedules will in most cases achieve a correct assessment of the patient's situation in time for effective therapy in many cases.

4 Follow-up of Malignant Lymphoma of the Thyroid

With this disease a similar situation exists as in the case of adeno-carcinoma of the thyroid: Several pathological entities are sometimes thrown into one pot, while in other places sophisticated classifications try to distinguish a considerable number of lymphoma types (Meissner, Warren 1969). Originally such tumors were called "lymphosarcomas" of the thyroid gland (Crile et al. 1955) and only in recent decades thyroidal manifestations of various systemic types of malignant lymphoma were described (Roberts, Howard 1963). Some authors were convinced only a few years ago that malignant thyroid lymphoma is an absolutely fatal disease with an expected life-span of 1–2 years (Oberdisse et al. 1980) but our group has much better results.

It certainly is essential for any follow-up program

a) to establish a correct diagnosis by histology, immunohistology, lymphocyte studies, whole body exams of the lymphatic system by ultrasound, CT-scanning, radiographs etc.
b) To decide on the basis of all the available diagnostic information whether the thyroid tumor is a local malignancy or just a special manifestation in systemic lymphatic malignancies (Maurer et al. 1979) and
c) possibly to review any initial TNM-stagings and/or pathological classifications according to the obtained findings.

If – e.g. – the removed tumor has to be considered as a thyroidal manifestation of generalized systemic lymphomata, treatment and follow-up will be chosen according to the guidelines developed in hematology and general on-

Table 48. Follow-up of patients with lymphosarcoma and other sarcomas

1st)	After surgery and radiotherapy according to staging results also chemotherapy, thyroid hormone.
2nd)	During 3 yrs. follow-up exams 4×/year with thyroid hormone medication (clinical exam, radiographs, ESR, blood count, T_4, TSH, tumor markers, CEA, Neopterin etc.).
3rd)	As in Table 43
4th)	As in Table 43
5th)	In case of tumor progression chemotherapy (radiotherapy).
6th)	Adapt programs to clinical course!

cology (Bayetta et al. 1981), taking into account also the specific type of neoplastic disease (Burke et al. 1977). If – on the other hand – the thyroid lesion is defined as a local "lymphosarcoma", no systemic chemotherapy, no staging interventions (Oberdisse et al. 1980) and only rarely large-field radiotherapy will be necessary (Harmer 1977). All these arguments justify the proposed follow-up program for this rare disease as shown in Table 28. It is obvious, that in such lesions a close cooperation between qualified pathologists, hematologists, radiotherapists and with the originally treating surgeon will be crucial if satisfactory long-term results are to be achieved. That such cures are possible is shown in the following case report:

Case W.P., male, 94.09.09.20

Since April 1973 pressure in the neck, palpitation in stress, somewhat tired, goiter known ~15 years, somewhat larger in recent months. Firm large goiter with single nodule on the right, nodule cold, chest films with residues after Tbc, otherwise normal, euthyroid. BSR and blood count normal. Cytology of thyroid: Pap. IV. Patient initially refusing surgery, finally accepting intervention which was carried out on November 14th, 1974 (near total thyroidectomy). Histology: Lymphosarcoma of the thyroid. Teleradiotherapy (60 Gy). Since then doing well with hypothyroidism as patient is not taking prescribed thyroid medication. No evidence of recurrence, metastases or systemic disease according to bone scan, sonography, radiograms, BSR and blood count (followed until November 1985).

Conclusions

At the end of this book it should be stated once again, that it does not present any exciting new scientific insights in thyroid cancer, but that it was written for practical purposes. The author tried hard, however, to include not only his own experiences (Riccabona 1986) but also the most significant older and recent reports on this peculiar disease, with reference to epidemiology, pathology, pathophysiology, diagnosis, treatment and follow-up. The long bibliography should enable interested readers to get special informations on a variety of special questions arising in the management of thyroid malignancies. The fact, that in the past 5 years at least 4 books (mostly congress reports) and more than 603 (!) scientific publications on thyroid cancer have been printed to the author's knowledge, that one recent surgical publication included 18 papers dealing with this disease (Langenbeck's Archiv 1985) and that a European Nuclear Medicine Congress report of 1984 (Vauramo, Schmidt 1985) contains 8 relevant presentations are proves that the topic retains considerable interest today and that it is impossible to quote every publication on the subject in this volume. We know of interesting work being done e.g. in India[1] by the groups of Kapur (New Delhi) and in Egypt by El-Haddad (Cairo), on theoretical and clinical aspects of thyroid cancer, but these sometimes fascinating studies have either not been published at all or in journals, which are difficult to obtain and to read in many parts of the world. The author suggested years ago (Riccabona 1980) that besides the very useful help of the UICC ("cancergrams") some international organization might provide ways and means to coordinate research on a world-wide level (e.g. WHO). You will also have noticed that we rarely come up with general answers or proposals for standard solutions in view of the manifold types of thyroid cancer. On the other hand we feel that with our knowledge and experience we can – perhaps – help to overcome the widespread diagnostic and therapeutic chaos that prevails in the management of thyroid cancer, which – as mentioned previously – now seems to increase after a period of relative stabilization.

We do not consider this book as the source of all wisdom for all time regarding thyroid cancer, it should rather serve as a sort of "common denominator" on the basis of which you can sort out your options and results and start plans for committed scientific and clinical research activities in the future.

---

[1] See also: Shah DH, Noronka OPD (eds) (1986) Thyroid Cancer: Radionuclides in Diagnosis etc. Rad Med Centre BARC, Bombay

Personally the author would be very happy if some hypotheses mentioned in the text could be documented convincingly or registered on the basis of solid data, if even better diagnostic and therapeutic approaches to the disease could be found and published in journals with a world-wide distribution, so that most doctors dealing with thyroid cancer would be informed. In this context I would like to remind you, that for a variety of reasons mentioned already "thyroid cancer" is a very different disease in many localities (e.g. in Zaire, in the United States or in Japan). The individual benefit for the patient must be the ultimate guideline for every medical approach, but we have to know which of the huge, frequently interesting and sometimes puzzling amounts of information on thyroid cancer are available. Only if we study carefully the literature on thyroid malignancies can we adapt our medical strategies to a given clinical situation. The effort is frequently rewarded by the patient's comments many years after appropriate treatment of thyroid malignancies:

Quote: patient P.S., fem. now 37 years, $T_3N_2M_0$, follicular carcinoma: "When I had my goiter operation in 1969 I thought that it would relieve me of a cosmetically disturbing tumor in my neck. When I heard that the tumor was malignant and that I had to have another intervention with a larger incision, that I should have treatment with radioactive iodine and several weeks of radiation therapy I was desperate. Your team helped me a lot to overcome this period. Now, as a happy, active and working woman I know, what has been done to me and I will always remain grateful to you all" (end of quote).

So, dealing with thyroid cancer we should keep the following points in mind:

a) "Primum nil nocere" (first of all do not harm).
b) Try to eliminate the malignant tumor as well as you can using your knowledge of all available techniques.
c) In cases with widespread disease try to control the tumor and relevant symptoms with appropriate therapy as long as possible.
d) Seek the active cooperation of the patient for treatment and follow-up and consider socio-economical circumstances and
e) keep abreast of new developments in basic sciences, diagnostic techniques and therapeutic approaches by intense study of the literature.

As you know, tuberculosis took a terrible death-toll in previous times, and thousands of people died and die from appendicitis all over the world every year. Considering the therapeutic potential for therapy of thyroid cancer today we have reason to hope that in a few decades the mortality of this malignant disease might dwindle to perhaps 10–20% and this is a promise for the future which justifies every relevant effort today.

References

Abrams HL, Spiro R, Goldstein N (1950) Metastases in carcinoma. Cancer 3:74

Ackerman NB, Marvin JF (1961) The use of radioactive phosphorus in the diagnosis of thyroid cancer. Radiology 77:793

Alexeiva-Figusch J, Van Gilse HA, Treutmiet RE (1978) Chemotherapy in carcinoma of the thyroid: retrospective and prospective. Ann Radiol 20:810

Attie JN, Khafif RA (1975) Preservation of parathyroid glands during total thyroidectomy. Amer J Surg 130:399

Balme H (1954) Metastatic carcinoma of thyroid successfully treated with thyroxine. Lancet 1:812

Bansi HW (1955) Krankheiten der Schilddrüse. In: Handbuch der Inneren Medizin. Springer, Berlin Göttingen Heidelberg, Vol VII/1, p 455

Bansi HW (1961) Schilddrüsendiagnostik mit Radiojod. In Schwiegk H, Turba F (ed) Künstliche radioaktive Isotope in Physiologie, Diagnostik und Therapie. Springer, Berlin Göttingen Heidelberg, Vol II, p 576

Barakat RM, Ingbar SH (1965) The effect of acute depletion of thyroid function in man. J clin Invest 44:1117

Barclay RS, McSwan N, Welsh TM (1957) Tracheal reconstruction without the use of grafts. Thorax 12:177

Baschieri L, Giani C, Taddei P, Lari R, Pinchera A (1981) Serum thyroglobulin as a marker of thyroid carcinoma. In: Andreoli M, Monaco F, Robbins J (ed) Advances in thyroid neoplasia. Field Educational Italia, Roma, p 189

Batz K, Hünig R, Nagel GA, Joos RA, Metzger V (1985) Therapie von Notfallsituationen und Komplikationen bei Tumorerkrankungen. In: Brunner KW, Nagel GA (ed) Internistische Krebstherapie. Springer, Berlin Heidelberg New York, p 159

Bauer R, Lauer O, Trappe A, Langhammer H, Schütz W, Lutilsky L, Stettmaier H, Pabst HW (1984) Clinically meaningful applications of NMR. Nucl Med, Suppl 21, p 75

Bauhofer G, Hausen A, Riccabona G (1978) Thyroxin und Trijodthyronin im Serum Euthyreoter nach Röntgenuntersuchungen mit jodhaltigen Kontrastmitteln. Münch Med Wschr 120:927

Bayetta E, Buzzoni R, Bonadonna G et al. (1981) Combined radiotherapy, chemotherapy (CVP vs. BACOP) in stage I–II diffuse non Hodgkin's lymphomas. In: Jones SE, Salmon SE (ed) Adjuvant therapy of cancer. III. Grune & Stratton, New York, p 107

Baylin SB (1974) Medullary carcinoma of the thyroid gland: Use of biochemical parameters in detection and surgical management of the tumor. Surg clin North Am 54:309

Beall AC, Harrington OB, Greenberg SD, Morris GC, Usher FC (1962) Tracheal replacement with heavy Marlex mesh: circumferential replacement of the cervical trachea. A.M.A. Arch Surg 84:390, 1962

Becker HD, Röher HD, Peitsch W, Wahl RA (1984) Chirurgie der malignen Struma. In: Becker HD, Heinze HD (ed) Maligne Schilddrüsentumoren. Springer, Berlin Heidelberg New York Tokyo, p 136

Beierwaltes WH (1978) Radioiodide in the therapy of thyroid carcinoma. In: Spencer RP (ed) Therapy in Nuclear Medicine. Grune & Stratton, New York San Francisco London

Benker G, Hackenberg K, Hoff HG, Seeber S, Ebke J, Windeck R, Reinwein D (1977) Zytostatische Kombinationsbehandlung metastasierender Schilddrüsenkarzinome mit Doxorubicin und Bleomycin. Dtsch med Wschr 102:1908

Benker G, Reinwein D (1983) Ergebnisse der Chemotherapie des Schilddrüsencarcinoms. Dtsch med Wschr 108:403
Benker G, Dabag S, Reinwein D, Seeber S (1984) Chemotherapie der Schilddrüsenkarzinome. In: Becker HD, Heinze HG (ed) Maligne Schilddrüsentumoren. Springer, Berlin Heidelberg New York Tokyo, p 187
Benua RS, Cicale NR, Sonnenberg MM, Rawson RW (1962) The relation of radioiodine dosimetry to results and complications in the treatment of metastatic thyroid cancer. Amer J Roentgenol 87:171
Benua RS, Yeh SDJ, Leeper RD (1982) Radioactive iodine therapy in thyroid cancer. J nucl Med 23:88
Berche Ch, Mach JP, Lumbroso JD, Langlais C, Parmentier C, Tubiana M (1982) Tomoscintigraphy for detecting gastrointestinal and medullary thyroid cancers: First clinical results using radiolabelled monoclonal antibodies against carcinoembryogenic antigen. Brit med J 285:1447
Boehme G (1983) Klinik der Sprach-, Sprech- und Stimmstörungen. Fischer, Stuttgart, 1983
Börner W (1976) Methoden zur Diagnostik des Solitärknotens der Schilddrüse. Med Welt 27:1611
Botsch H, Schulz E, Lochner B (1979) Serum-Thyreoglobulinbestimmung zur Verlaufskontrolle bei Schilddrüsenkarzinom-Patienten. Dtsch med Wschr 104:1072
Boyden SV (1951) The adsorption of proteins on erythrocytes treated with tannic acid and subsequent haemagglutination by antiprotein sera. J exp Med 93:107
Breitner B (1960) Chirurgische Operationslehre. Urban & Schwarzenberg, Vienna, Suppl Vol IX
Brill AB (1982) Low level radiation effects: A fact book. Soc Nucl Med, New York
Buell U, Niendorf HP, Kazner E, Lanksch W, Wilske J, Steinhoff H, Jahr H (1978) Computerized transaxial tomography and cerebral serial scintigraphy in intracranial tumors. J nucl Med 19:476
Burke JS, Butler JJ, Fuller LM (1977) Malignant lymphomas of the thyroid: A clinical pathological study of 35 patients including ultrastructural observations. Cancer 38:1587
Busnardo B, Bui D, Girelli ME, Casara D (1981) Rapid suppression of TSH-secretion using an optimal saturation regimen of thyroid hormones in patients with thyroid cancer. In: Andreoli M, Monaco F, Robbins J (ed) Advances in thyroid neoplasia. Field Educational Italia, Roma, p 341
Busnardo B, Girelli ME, Pelizzo MR, Zorat PL, De Besi P, Eccher C (1983) Different diagnostic significance of carcinoembryonic antigen vs. calcitonin as tumor marker of medullary thyroid carcinoma. Acta endocrinol. (Kbh.) Suppl. 252, p 57
Byar DP, Green SB, Dor P, Williams ED, Colon J, van Gilse HA, Mayer M, Sylvester RJ, van Glabbcke M (1979) A prognostic index for thyroid carcinoma. A study of the EORTC thyroid cancer cooperative group. Europ J Cancer 15:1033
Cabanne F, Gerard-Marchant R, Heimann R, Williams ED (1974) Tumeurs malignes du corps thyroide: Problèmes de diagnostique histopathologique. Ann anat path 19:129
Calmette C, Moukhtar MS, Millaud G (1978) Plasma carcinoembryonic antigen versus plasma calcitonin in the diagnosis of the thyroid. Cancer immunol Immunother 4:251
Carr DH, Brown J, Leung AWL, Pennock JM (1984) Iron and gadolinium chelates as contrast agents in NMR imaging: Preliminary studies. J Comput Assist Tomogr 8:385
Clark OH (1981) TSH suppression in the management of thyroid nodules and thyroid cancer. World J Surg 5:39
Clark OH (1982) Total thyroidectomy. The treatment of choice for patients with differentiated thyroid cancer. Ann Surg 196:361
Cohen SL, Grahame-Smith D, MacIntyre I, Walker JG (1973) Alcohol-stimulated calcitonin release in medullary carcinoma of the thyroid. Lancet II:1172
Cope O (1962) Personal communication
Crile G jr, Hazard JB, Dinsmore RS (1948) Carcinoma of the thyroid gland with special reference to the clinico-pathological classification. Trans Amer Goiter Ass, p 159
Crile G (1955) Treatment of cancer of the thyroid with desiccated thyroid. Cleveland Clin Quart 22:161
DeGroot LJ, Stanbury JB (1975) The thyroid and its diseases. Wiley & Sons, New York London Sydney Toronto

DeGroot LJ, Hoye K, Refetoff S, van Herle AJ, Asteris GI, Rochmann H (1977) Serum antigens and antibodies in the diagnosis of thyroid cancer. J clin Endocrin 45:1220

Doll R (1969) Summarizing statement on results of treatment. In: Hedinger Chr (ed) Thyroid cancer. Springer, Berlin Heidelberg New York, p 309

Droese M (1979) Aspirationscytologie der Schilddrüse. Schattauer, Stuttgart

Dunn JT, Ray SC (1973) Changes in iodine metabolism and thyroglobulin structure in metastatic follicular carcinoma of the thyroid with hyperthyroidism. J clin Endocrin 36:1088

Durie BGM (1981) High risk thyroid cancer: Prolonged survival with early multimodality therapy. Cancer clin Trials 4:67

Ebers G (1875) Papyros Ebers. Leipzig, Vol. 1–2

Edis AJ, Ayala LA, Egdahl RH (1975) Surgery of the thyroid. In: Manual of endocrine surgery. Springer, Berlin Heidelberg New York

Edmonds ChJ, Kermoda JC (in press) Radioiodine concentration by differentiated thyroid cancers in relation to TSH cell membrane receptors and thyroglobulin secretion. Proc. 1st European Symp. Thyroid Cancer. Elsevier, Amsterdam

Ell PJ (1980) Radioisotope single photon tomography, clinical applications. Nucl Med, Schattauer, Stuttgart New York, Suppl 17, p 104

Ellenberg AH, Goldman L, Gordan GS, Lindsay S (1962) Thyroid carcinoma in patients with hyperparathyroidism. Surgery 51:708

Ellis SM, Ekins R (1973) The radioimmunoassay of free T_3 and T_4 concentration in serum. Proc Soc Endocrinol 14:59

Emrich D (1979) Nuklearmedizinische Funktionsdiagnostik und Therapie. Thieme, Stuttgart

Esselstyn CB (1983) Individualizing the extent of surgery for thyroid cancer: A reappraisal. In: Thompson NW, Vinik AI (ed) Endocrine surgery update. Grune & Stratton, New York London, p 67

Fairweather DS, Bradwell AR, Watson-Janees SF, Dykes PW, Chandler S, Hoffenberg R (1983) Detection of thyroid tumors using radiolabelled anti-thyroglobulin. Clin Endocrinol 18:563

Fasching W (1984) Manual der chirurgischen Krebstherapie. Facultas Ed. Vienna

Fassbender HG (1956) Pathologische Anatomie der endokrinen Drüsen. A: Die Schilddrüse. In: Staemmler M (ed) Lehrbuch der speziellen pathologischen Anatomie. DeGruyter, Berlin 11th & 12th ed., Vol 1/2

Feine U, Grann H, Huebener H, Rücker HC (1979) Vergleichende Untersuchungen zur Szintigraphie, Transmissionscomputertomographie und Ultraschalltomographie (B-Scan) von Leber und Milz. Nucl Med, Schattauer, Stuttgart New York, Suppl 17, p 155

Feine U, zum Winkel K (1980) Nuklearmedizin – szintigraphische Diagnostik. Thieme, Stuttgart New York

Forester CF (1963) Coma in myxedema. Report of a case and review of the world literature. Arch intern Med III:734

Frank Th (1980) Ultraschall in der Schilddrüsendiagnostik. Röntgen Bl 33:386

Fuchsig P, Bruniak R, Schnayder K (1963) Über den Strömungswiderstand in normalen und pathologischen Tracheen. Klin Med 18:174

Fuchsig P, Keminger K (1972) Chirurgie der Schilddrüse und der Nebenschilddrüse. In: Naumann HH (ed) Kopf- und Halschirurgie. Thieme, Stuttgart, Vol I

Gadian DG (1982) In: Nuclear magnetic resonance and it's application to living systems. Clarendon Press, Oxford

Galvan G (1970) Feinnadelpunktion und Zytodiagnostik kalter Strumaknoten im Strumaendemiegebiet. Dtsch med Wschr 95:1631

Galvan G (1983) The value of the aspiration biopsy cytology for the diagnosis of thyroid malignancies. Acta endocrinol (Kbh), Suppl. 252, p 55

Galvan G, Prates B, Thurner J, Steiner H (1984) Strumacysten und Malignität. Nucl Med Suppl 20, Schattauer, Stuttgart New York, p 792

Geißl G, Heinze HG, Pickardt CR (1977) TSH-Spiegel nach Schilddrüsenhormonentzug bei athyreoten Schilddrüsenkarzinompatienten. Münchn med Wschr 119:697

Gemsenjäger E (1978) Zur chirurgischen Therapie der differenzierten Schilddrüsenkarzinome. Dtsch med Wschr 103:749

Gerard-Marchant R (1977) The classification of thyroid cancers according to the TNM system. Ann Radiol 20:700

Glanzmann CH, Horst W (1979) Behandlung und Prognose des follikulären und papillären Schilddrüsenkarzinoms. Erfahrungen mit kombinierter chirurgisch-radiologischer Therapie bei 200 Patienten in dem Zeitraum 1963 bis 1977. Strahlentherapie 155:151

Goltzmann D, Potts JI, Ridgway EC, Maloff F (1974) Calcitonin as a tumor marker. New Engl J Med 290:1035

Granier AM, Houcke M, Proye C, Delobells A, Borniere C (in press) Le diagnostic cytologique du carcinome medullaire de la thyroide. In: Proc. 1st European Symp. on thyroid cancer. Elsevier, Amsterdam New York

Grant S, Luttrell V, Reeve T et al. (1984) Thyroglobulin may be undetectable in the serum of patients with metastatic secondary to differentiated thyroid carcinoma: Follow-up of differentiated thyroid carcinoma. Cancer 54:1625

Grillo C (1968) Resektion und Rekonstruktion der Trachea. Langenbecks Arch klin Chir 322:869

Grunicke H (1980) Nuklearmedizin und in vitro Methoden (klinisch-chemische Aspekte). Nucl Med, Suppl 17, p 767

Guilloteau D, Baulieu JL, Besuard JC (1985) Medullary-thyroid-carcinoma imaging in an animal model: use of radiolabeled anticalcitonin F $(ab')_2$ and meta-iodobenzyl-guanidine. Europ J nucl Med 11:198

Hall R, Amos J, Ormston BJ (1971) Radioimmunoassays for serum thyrotropin. Brit med J I/582

Halnan KE (1975) The non-surgical treatment of thyroid cancer. Brit J Surg 62:769

Halnan KE (1982) The treatment of cancer. Chapman & Hall, London

Hamberger JI, Miller JM (1981) Controversies in clinical thyroidology. Springer, New York Heidelberg Berlin

Hamlin E, Vickery AL (1956) Needle biopsy of the thyroid gland. New Engl J Med 254:742

Harada T, Shimaoka K, Mimura T, Ito K (1981) Chemotherapy of thyroid cancer. In: Andreoli M, Monaco F, Robbins J (ed) Advances in thyroid neoplasia. Field Educational Italia, Roma, p 347

Harmer CL (1977) External beam radiotherapy for thyroid cancer. Ann Radiol. 20:791

Heinze HG (1984) Nachsorge und Nachkontrolle bei Patienten mit malignen Schilddrüsentumoren. In: Becker HD, Heinze HG (ed) Maligne Schilddrüsentumoren. Springer, Berlin Heidelberg New York Tokyo, p 290

Hellman DE, Durie BGM, Woolenden JM, Karlehner M (1980) Multidisciplinary management of carcinoma of the thyroid. Ariz Med 37:19

Hermann HJ, Kimmig B, Strumpf HP, Hufner M (1985) Computertomographie in der Nachsorge des differenzierten Schilddrüsenkarzinoms. Röntgenblätter 38:159

Hickey RC, Samaan NA (1975) Human parathyroid autotransplantation. Arch Surg 110:892

Hoffer PB, Gottschalk A, Refetoff S (1972) Thyroid scanning techniques: The old and the new. Curr Prob Radiol 2:5

Hoffman DP, Surks MI, Oppenheimer JH, Weitzmann DE (1977) Response to thyrotropin releasing hormone: An objective criterion for the adequacy of thyrotropin suppression therapy. J Clin Endocrinol Metab 44:892

Horn RC (jr) (1955) The pathologic physiology of carcinoma of the thyroid. Surg Clin N Amer 35:1669

Horst W (1961) Radiojod in Diagnostik und Therapie der Schilddrüsenneoplasmen. In: Künstliche radioaktive Isotope in Physiologie, Diagnostik und Therapie. Springer, Berlin Göttingen Heidelberg, Vol II, p 886

Horst W (1985) Schilddrüsenkrebs. In: Gross R, Schmidt CG (ed) Klinische Onkologie. Thieme, Stuttgart New York, 38:1

Huber P (1956) Die Struma maligna. Strahlentherapie, Sonderbd. 34:100

Huber P (1958) Diagnostische Irrtümer und Behandlungsfehler bei Schilddrüsenerkrankungen. Chir Praxis 1:89

Huber P, Riccabona G (1967) Diagnostik und Therapie der Schilddrüsenerkrankungen vom Gesichtspunkt des Chirurgen aus. In: Klinische Chirurgie für die Praxis. Thieme, Stuttgart, p 145

Huber P (1973) Eingriffe am Hals. In: Breitner B (ed) Chirurgische Operationslehre. Erg Beitrg Vol II. Urban & Schwarzenberg, Wien, p 46

Hüfner M, Munzinger H, Papke H, Barwick D, Balmer F, Schenk P, Röher D (1975) Prinzipien der Hormonsubstitution bei thyreoidektomierten Schilddrüsen-Karzinompatienten. Radiologe 15:245

Hugl H, Unterkircher S, Kloss K, Riccabona G (1978) Die Bedeutung der dynamisch-statischen Hirnszintigraphie für die Erfassung von Gehirntumorrezidiven. Nucl Med, Suppl 16. Schattauer, Stuttgart New York, p 447

Hundeshagen H (1980) In: Diethelm L, Henck F, Olsson O, Vieten H, Zuppinger A (ed) Handbuch der medizinischen Radiologie. Springer, Berlin Heidelberg New York Tokyo, Vol 15, part 1 A

Hundeshagen H (1983) Postoperative diagnosis and therapy of thyroid malignomas by nuclear medicine. Acta endocrinol (Kbh) 102, Suppl 252, p 81

Hundeshagen H (1984) Gegenwärtiger Stand und zukünftige Entwicklung der NMR-Tomographie. Nucl Med Suppl 21, p 63

Jaffiol C, Lamargue JL, Augustin I, Ronanet JP, Collet H, Longchamp Y, Baldet L, Hercot O, Rossi M, Pujol J (in press) Thyroid imaging for the diagnosis and the posttherapeutic control of thyroid carcinoma. Proc 1st European Symposium on Thyroid Cancer. Elsevier, Amsterdam

Iida F, Yonekura M, Miyakawa M (1969) Study of intraglandular dissemination of thyroid cancer. Cancer 24:764

Illich (1976) Limits to Medicine. Boyers Marion, London 1976

Joumans J (1982) Neurological Surgery. Saunders & Roe, Philadelphia, Vol VI

Ishikawa H, Hamada S (1976) Association of medullary carcinoma of the thyroid with carcino-embryonic antigen. Brit J Cancer 34:111

Izumi M, Larsen PR (1978) Correlation of sequential changes in serum thyroglobulin, triiodothyronine and thyroxine in patients with Graves' disease and subacute thyroiditis. Metabolism 27:449

Kagan AR, Nussbaum H, Chan P, Leoni R (1974) Thyroid carcinoma: is postoperative external irradiation indicated? Oncology 29:401

Kaul A, Roedler D (1977) Strahlenschutz in der Nuklearmedizin: Grundlagen und Methoden. In Lorenz WJ (ed) Medizinische Physik. Hüthig, Heidelberg, Vol 1, p 341

Keminger K (1964) Zur radikalen Lymphknotenexstirpation bei Schilddrüsenmalignomen. Klin Med 19:310

King WLM, Pemberton JJ (1942) So-called lateral aberrant thyroid tumors. Surg Gynec Obstet 74:991

Klein E, Heinze BG, Hoffmann G, Reinwein D, Schneider C (1974) Therapie der Schilddrüsenmalignome. Dtsch med Wschr 101:835

Klein E, Reinwein D (1978) Klinische Endokrinologie. Schattauer, Stuttgart New York

Koch O, Uhlenbruck G, Gross R (1984) Marker, Malignome und monoklonale Antikörper. Dtsch Ärztebl 81:1

Kohn LD, Meldolesi MF, Aloj SM, Vitti P, Valente WA, Lacetti P, Cohen JL, Dianzani U, Grollmann EF (1981) A molecular model of the thyrotropin receptor: experimental and human thyroid tumors with relevant defects. In: Andreoli M, Monaco F, Robbins J (ed) Advances in thyroid neoplasia. Field Educational Italia, Roma, p 23

Kremkan FW (1980) Diagnostic ultrasound, physical principles and exercises. Grune & Stratton, New York

La France ND, Dorner MW, Larson S et al. (1985) Diagnostische Anwendung monoklonaler Antikörper. Dtsch med Wschr 110:651

Lamberg BA, Rantanen M, Saarinen P (1977) Choosing thyroxine dose after treatment of thyroid cancer. Lancet 2:1290

Langenbecks Arch f Chir (1985) Vol 366

Leisner B, Degelmann G, Dirr W, Kaintz W, Büll U, Langhammer H, Lissner J, Pabst HW (1982) Behandlungsergebnisse bei Struma maligna 1960–1980. Stellenwert der perkutanen Nachbestrahlung bei differenzierten Karzinomen. Dtsch med Wschr 107:1702

Lenzhofer R, Dudczak R, Dittrich C, Gumbold G, Moser K, Spitzy KH (1983) Überwachung der Herzfunktion bei Doxorubicintherapie des metastasierten Mammakarzinoms. Dtsch med Wschr 108:771

Lindsay S, Dailey ME (1965) Malignant lymphoma of the thyroid gland and its relation to Hashimoto Disease. J clin endocrin 15:1332

Löffler W, Oppelt A (1981) Physical principles of NMR-Tomography. Europ J Radiol 1:338
Maier R (1984) Ultraschalldiagnostik der Schilddrüse. Schattauer, Stuttgart New York
Martz G (1968) Die hormonale Therapie maligner Tumoren. Springer, Berlin Heidelberg New York
Maurer R, Taylor CR, Terry R, Lukes RJ (1979) Non Hodgkin lymphomas of the thyroid. A clinico-pathological review of 29 cases and an immunoperoxydase method. Virchow's Arch Pathol Anat 383:293
McAfee JG, Stern AS, Fueger GF, Baggish MS, Holgman GB, Zolle I (1964) ^{99m}Tc labeled serum albumin for scintillation scanning of the placenta. J nucl Med 5:936
Means JH, DeGroot LJ, Stanbury JB (1963) The thyroid and its diseases. McGraw-Hill, New York Toronto London
Meighan JW, Dworkin HJ (1969) Failure to detect ^{131}I positive thyroid metastases with ^{99m}Tc. J Nucl Med 11:173
Meissner WA, Lahey FH (1948) Cancer of the thyroid in a thyroid clinic. J clin Endocrin 8:749
Meissner WA, Warren S (1969) Lymphoma of the thyroid. In: Tumors of the thyroid gland. Armed Forces Institute of Path., Washington, 2nd series, fasc 14, p 122
Meyer R (1971) Behandlung der Trachealstenosen. Arch klin exp. Ohr-Nas- u Kehlk-Heilk 199:292
Miller JM, Hamberger JI (1965) The thyroid scintigram I. The hot nodule. Radiology 84:66
Miyata Y, Sasaki T, Takaya K, Taguchi Y. New approach for diagnosis of malignant goiter with nuclear magnetic resonance. In: "Frontiers in Thyroidology". Plenum, New York London, 1986, Vol 2, p 1303
Naumann HH (1972) Kopf- und Halschirurgie. Thieme, Stuttgart Vol I
Nishiyama RH, Ludwig GK, Thompson NL (1977) The prevalence of small papillary thyroid carcinomas in 100 consecutive necropsies in an American population. In: DeGroot LJ (ed) Radiation associated thyroid carcinoma. Grune & Stratton, New York, p 123
Nittner K (1980) Möglichkeiten der neurochirurgischen Schmerzbeeinflussung. Fortschr Neurol Psych 48:571
Olen E, Klinck GH (1965) The association of hyperthyroidism and thyroid cancer. In: Cassano C, Andreoli M (ed) Thyroid research. Academic Press, New York London, p 1023
Orvoine RH, Cantin M, Garzon S, Billick RC, Stephens H, Strykowsky H (1983) Dedifferentiation of a transplantable papillary thyroid carcinoma over a 15-year period. Cancer 52:1720
Ota H, Yamamoto K, Endo K, Mori T, Hamanaka D, Shimazu A, Ikekubo K, Makimoto K, Iida Y, Konishi J, Morita R, Hata N, Horiuchi K, Yokoyama A, Torizuka K, Kuma K (1984) A new imaging agent for medullary carcinoma of the thyroid. J nucl Med 25:323
Parthmore JG, Bronzert D, Roberts G, Deftos LJ (1974) A short calcium infusion in the diagnosis of medullary thyroid carcinoma. J clin Endocrinol 39:108
Patton JA, Hallifield JW, Brill AB, Lee GS, Patton DD (1976) Differentiation between malignant and benign solitary thyroid nodules by fluorescent scanning. J nucl Med 17:17
Peiper HJ, Becker HD, Peitsch W (1980) Indikationen und operative Strategie beim Schilddrüsencarcinom. In: Schauer A (ed) Zur Diagnostik und Therapie von Schilddrüsentumoren. Schattauer, Stuttgart, p 79
Pemberton JJ (1939) Malignant lesions of thyroid gland: review of 774 cases. Surg Gynec Obstet 69:417
Persson PS (1967) Cytodiagnosis of thyroiditis. Acta med Scand Suppl 483
Pezzino V, Vigneri R, Squatrito S, Filetti S, Camus M, Polose P (1978) Increased serum thyroglobulin levels in patients with nontoxic goiter. J clin Endocrin Metab 46:653
Pfannenstiel P, Andrews GA, Brown DW (1965) Congenital hypothyroidism from intrauterine ^{131}I-damage. In: Current topics in thyroid research. Academic Press, New York London, p 749
Pickardt CR (1984) Hormontherapie des Schilddrüsenmalignoms. In: Becker HD, Heinze HG (ed) Maligne Schilddrüsentumoren. Springer, Berlin Heidelberg New York Tokyo, p 177
Pochin EE (1971) Radioiodine therapy of thyroid cancer. Semin nucl Med 1:503
Pohl G, Boeckl O, Galvan G, Salis-Samaden R, Steiner H, Thurner J (1977) Konkordantes medulläres Schilddrüsenkarzinom bei eineiigen Zwillingen mit diskordantem Phäochromocytom (Sipple Syndrom). Wiener klin Wschr 89:481
Portmann EV (1941) Experiences in the treatment of the malignant tumors of the thyroid gland. Amer J Roentgenol 46:46

Poster DS, Bruno S, Pina K, Catane R (1981) Current status of chemotherapy in the treatment of advanced carcinoma of the thyroid gland. Cancer clin Trials 4:301
Rall JE, Miller WN, Forster CG, Peacock WC, Rawson RW (1951) The use of thiouracil in the treatment of metastatic carcinoma of the thyroid with radioiodine. J clin Endocrinol 11:1273
Reiners Chr (1981) Spezifische und unspezifische Tumormarker beim Schilddrüsenkarzinom etc. Tumor-Diagnostik 2:199
Reiners Chr (1983) Serum thyroglobulin as a substitution of ^{131}I-scans in follow-up of differentiated thyroid cancer? Acta endocrinol. (Kbh), Suppl 252, p 66
Reinwein D, Klein E (1982) Diminished thyroid hormone formation. Schattauer, Stuttgart New York
Riccabona G (1972) Die endemische Struma. Urban & Schwarzenberg, München Berlin Wien
Riccabona G (1973) Schilddrüse. In: Chirurgie der Gegenwart. Urban & Schwarzenberg, München Berlin Wien, Vol VII, p 1
Riccabona G (1977) Anwendung von Radionukliden bei der Diagnose und Therapie von Schilddrüsenerkrankungen. Wien med Wschr 127:97
Riccabona G (1978) Diagnostik und Therapie der Struma maligna. Therapiewoche 28:9874
Riccabona G (1979) Intracavitäre Isotopentherapie. Nucl Med Suppl 16, p 698
Riccabona G (1980) Thyroid cancer and endemic goiter. In: Stanbury JB, Hetzel BS (ed) Endemic goiter and endemic cretinism. J. Wiley & Sons, New York Chichester Brisbane Toronto, p 333
Riccabona G, Unterkircher S (1981) Zur Betreuung von Patienten mit maligner Struma. Z Allg Med 57:1906
Riccabona G (1982) Epidemiologie der Struma maligna. Schweiz Rundschau Med (Praxis) 13:523
Riccabona G (1984) Therapy with radionuclides. Nuklearmedizin Suppl 20. Schattauer, Stuttgart New York, p 910
Riccabona G. Thyroid cancer and other surgical problems in areas of endemic goiter. In: Dunn JT, Pretell E (ed) Endemic goiter and endemic cretinism. PAHO scientific publ. No 502, 1986, p 68
Riccabona G (1986) Treatment of pleural and peritoneal carcinosis with radioactive colloids. In: Winkler C (ed) Nuclear medicine in clinical oncology. Springer, Berlin Heidelberg, p 362
Riccabona G, Benesovsky M (1966) Biological changes in the course of metastatic carcinoma of the thyroid and their significance for therapy. Intern Surgery 45:88
Roberts TW, Howard RG (1963) Primary Hodgkin's disease of the thyroid. Ann Surg 157:625
Rösler H, Moser M (1984) Schwangerschaft nach hochdosierter Radiojodtherapie. Nucl Med, Suppl 20, p 920
Rosvoll RV, Winship T (1965) Thyroid carcinoma and pregnancy. In: Current topics in thyroid research. Academic Press, New York London, p 1042
Roy-Camille R, Savoie JC, Gagne G, Mazel Ch (in press) Traitement des metastases osseuses des cancers thyroidiens. Proc. 1st European Symposium on thyroid cancer, Elsevier, Amsterdam
Ruckensteiner E (1963) Die Röntgenuntersuchung bei Strumen. Wien med Wschr 113:817
Russell WO, Ibanez ML, Clark RL, White EC (1963) Thyroid carcinoma. Cancer 36:553
Salvatore M, Mansi L (1981) ^{201}Thallium scan as a marker for thyroid neoplasia. In: Andreoli M, Monaco F, Robbins J (ed) Advances in thyroid neoplasia. Field educational Italia, Roma, p 225
Samonigg H, Leb G, Goebel R, Fereberger W, Biffl E (1983) Aclacinomycin-A, a new cytostatic agent in the treatment of thyroid carcinoma. Acta endocrinol (Kbh), Suppl 252, p 77
Samuels BI (1972) Thermography: a valuable tool in the detection of thyroid disease. Radiology 102:59
Schatz H, Grebe SF, Horn F, Müller H (1983) Thyroglobulin and thyroid carcinoma: Comparison between thyroglobulin levels on and off T_4, 2 mCi ^{131}I-scans and post-therapeutic scans. Acta endocrinol (Kbh), Suppl 252, p 65
Schauer A (1984) Pathogenese und pathologische Anatomie. In: Becker HD, Heinze HG (ed) Maligne Schilddrüsentumoren. Springer, Berlin Heidelberg New York Tokyo, p 2

Schicha H, Facorr U, Schurmbrand P, Schreivogel P, Emrich D (1980) Frequency of iodine contamination in a thyroid clinic. J Molecul Med 4:177
Schlorhaufer W (1986) Personal communication
Schlumberger M, van Herle AJ, Di Paola R, Viguel A, Di Paola M, Kahn E, Tubiana M (1983) In vivo localization of radiolabeled antibodies to rat thyroglobulin in the I-IC_2 rat thyroid transplantable tumor. Acta endocrinol (Kbh) Suppl 252, 43
Schneekloth F, Frank T, Albers G (1983) Ultraschalltomographie abdomineller Organe und der Schilddrüse. Enke, Stuttgart
Schwarz K, Scriba PC (1969) Endokrinologie für die Praxis. Lehmann, München, Vol I
Schwarzrock R, Müller St, Schober O, Hundeshagen H (1983) Bedeutung der Sonographie für die Diagnose der Schilddrüsenmalignome. Akt Endokr Stoffw, 4:107
Sedgwick CE (1974) Surgery of the thyroid gland. Saunders, Philadelphia London Toronto
Seidlin SM, Oshry E, Yalow AA (1948) Spontaneous and experimentally induced uptake of radioactive iodine in metastases from thyroid carcinoma: A preliminary report. J clin Endocrin 8:423
Seidlin SM, Rossman J, Oshry E, Siegel E (1949) Radioiodine therapy of metastases from carcinoma of the thyroid (A six years progress report). J clin Endocrinol 9:1122
Sgalitzer M, Stöhr W (1924) Röntgenuntersuchung der Luftröhre unter besonderer Berücksichtigung der Tracheomalazie. Fortschr Röntgenstr 32:247
Shafer RB, Tully TE (1974) Thyroid carcinoma presenting as an isolated bone cyst. J nucl Med 15:50
Sheperd PS, Lazarus CR, Mistry RD et al. (1985) Detection of thyroid tumor using a monoclonal ^{123}I-anti-human thyroglobulin antibody. Europ J Nucl Med 10:291
Shimaoka K (1980) Adjunctive management of thyroid cancer: Chemotherapy. J Surg Oncol 15:283
Shimaoka K, Sokal JE, Pickren W (1962) Metastatic neoplasms in the thyroid gland. Cancer 15:557
Siegel EP, Hart HE, Brothers M, Spencer H, Laszlo D (1956) Radio-Yttrium (^{90}Y) for the palliative treatment of effusions due to malignancy. JAMA 161:499
Sipple JH (1961) Association of phaeochromocytoma with carcinoma of the thyroid gland. Am J Med 31:163
Snyder J, Gorman C, Scanlon P (1983) Thyroid remnant ablation: Questionable pursuit of an all ill-defined goal? J Nucl Med 24:659
Spencer RP (1978) Therapy in Nuclear Medicine. Grune & Stratton, New York San Francisco London
Spiessl B, Hermanek P, Scheibe D (1982) TNM-Atlas. Springer, Berlin Heidelberg
Stanbury JB, Brownell GL, Riggs DS, Perinetti H, Itoiz J, del Castillo EB (1954) Endemic goiter. Harvard University Press, Cambridge, Mass
Steiner H, Salis-Samaden R (1966) Strahlenbehandlung und Operabilität maligner Strumen. Bruns Beitr klin Chir 213:188
Stieve FE (1976) Das Risiko der Gefährdung bei der Anwendung ionisierender Strahlung in der Medizin im Vergleich zu anderen Anwendungen. In: Strahlenschutz in Forschung und Praxis. Thieme, Stuttgart, Vol 16, p 203
Subramanian G, McAfee IG, Blair RJ, Kallfelz FA, Thomas FD (1975) Technetium ^{99m}Methylene Diphosphonate – a superior agent for skeletal imaging: Comparison with other technetium complexes. J Nucl Med 16:744
Suen KC, Wood WS, Syed AA, Quenville NF, Clement PB (1978) Role of imprint cytology in intraoperative diagnosis: value and limitations. J clin Pathol. 31:328
Svyatuklinan OV, Lazarev NI, Lemkova YT (1969) Endocrine aspects of thyroid cancer therapy. In: Hedinger Chr (ed) Thyroid cancer. Springer, Berlin Heidelberg New York, p 266
Syrota A, Duquesney N, Kellershohn C (1982) Positron emission tomographic evaluation of the pancreas. Nucl Med Suppl 19, p 217
Taylor S, Steiner W, Egdahl HR, Röher HD (1976) Diagnosis and treatment of thyroid cancer. Langenbecks Arch Chir 343:1
Taylor S, Al-Wattar K (1980) Surgical management. In: Duncan W (ed) Thyroid Cancer. Springer, Berlin Heidelberg New York, p 102

Taylor KJW, Carpenter DA, Barrett JJ (1974) Gray-scale ultrasonography in the diagnosis of thyroid swellings. J clin Ultrasound 2:327
Tejero-Vidal J (1979) Recent advances in scintigraphy of the central nervous system. Nucl Med Suppl 16, Schattauer, Stuttgart New York, p 254
Thijs LJ (1971) Diagnostic ultrasound in clinical thyroid investigation. J clin Endocrinol & Metab 32:709
Thomas CG (1958) The use of L-triiodothyronine as a pituitary depressant in the management of thyroid cancer. Surg Gynec Obstet 106:137
Thompson NW, Olsen WR, Hoffmann GL (1973) The continuing development of the technique of thyroidectomy. Surgery 73:913
Thompson NW, Vinik AI (1983) Endocrine surgery update. Grune & Stratton, New York London
Tollefsen HR, Shak JP, Huvos AG (1972) Papillary carcinoma of the thyroid. Recurrence in the thyroid gland after initial surgical treatment. Amer J Surg 124:468
Tubiana M (1982) Thyroid cancer. In: Beckers Chr (ed) Thyroid diseases. Pergamon, Oxford, p 187
Tubiana M, Charbord P, Zukersztein W, Sazzazick D, Fontaine F, Parmentier C (1977) The role of radiotherapy and radioactive iodine in the treatment of thyroid cancer without metastases. Ann Radiol 20:801
UICC (1976) TNM-Klassifizierung der malignen Tumoren. 2nd Ed. Springer, Berlin
UICC (1979) TNM-Klassifikation der malignen Tumoren. 3rd Ed., Springer, Berlin
Valenta L (1966) Metastatic thyroid carcinoma in man concentrating iodine without organification. J clin Endocrinol Metab 26:1317
Van Herle AJ, Uller RP (1975) Elevated serum thyroglobulin: a marker of metastasis in differentiated thyroid carcinoma. J clin Invest 56:272
Vauramo E, Schmidt HAE (1984) Nuklearmedizin in Forschung und Praxis. Nukl Med Suppl 21
Veith FJ, Gupta SK, Samson RH et al. (1981) Progress in limb salvage by reconstructive arterial surgery combined with new or improved adjunctive measures. Ann Surg 194:386
Vider M, DeLand F, Mercuyama Y (1976) Loculation as a contraindication to intracavitary ^{32}P chromic phosphate therapy. J Nucl Med 17:150
Vogl S, Ohmma T, Perloff M, Holland JF (1976) Combination therapy with adriamycin and cis-diamine-dichloroplatinum in patients with neoplastic diseases. Cancer 38:21
Wagner HN (1974) Nuclear Medicine. HP Publ Co, New York
Walfish PG, Hazani E, Strawbridge HTG, Miskui M, Rosen IB (1977) Combined ultrasound and needle aspiration cytology in the assessment and management of hypofunctioning thyroid nodule. Ann Int Med 87:270
Walther HE (1948) Krebsmetastasen. Schwabe, Basel
Weeks I, Woodhead JS (1984) Chemiluminescent acridium esters as labels in immunoassay. In: Kricka LJ et al. (ed) Analytical applications of bioluminescence and chemiluminescence. Academic Press, London, p 185
Weissel M, Höfer R (1983) Carcinoembryonic antigen (CEA) in thyroid cancer. Acta endocrinol (Kbh), Suppl 252, p 60
Weissel M, Bergmann H, Höfer R (1984) Optimiertes Nachsorgeschema bei differenzierten Schilddrüsenkarzinomen. Kongr Ber 25. Jahrestagung Österr. Ges f Chir, Graz
Wells PNT (1977) Biomedical Ultrasonics. Academic Press, London
Wells SA, Ontjes DA, Cooper CW, Hennessy JF, Ellis GJ, McPherson HT, Sabiston DC (1975) The early diagnosis of medullary carcinoma of the thyroid gland in patients with multiple neoplasia type II. Ann Surg 182:360
Wells SA, Baylin SB, Linehan WM, Farrel RE, Cox EB, Cooper CW (1978) Provocative agents and the diagnosis of medullary carcinoma of the thyroid gland. Ann Surg 188:139
Wenzel KW, Meinhold H (1974) Evidence of lower toxicity during thyroxine suppression after a single 3 mg l-thyroxine dose. Comparison to the classical l-triiodothyronine test for thyroid suppressibility. J clin Endocrinol 38:890
Werner S (1969) Classification of thyroid disease. J clin Endocrinol 29:860
Wieland DM, Wu JL, Brown LE, Mangner TJ, Swanson DP, Beierwaltes WH (1980) Radiolabled adrenergic neuron blocking agents: adrenomedullary imaging with ^{131}I-iodobenzylguanidine. J Nucl Med 21:349

Williams ED (1979) Medullary carcinoma of the thyroid. In: DeGroot LJ (ed) Endocrinology. Vol 2. Grune & Stratton, New York, p 777

Wilson J (1921) Malignant tumors of the thyroid. Ann Surg 74

Winchell HS, Sanchez PD, Watanabe CK, Hollander L, Anger HO, McRae J, Hayes RL, Edwards LC (1970) Visualization of tumors using ^{67}Ga-citrate and the Anger whole body scanner, scintillation camera and tomographic scanner. J Nucl Med 11:459

Wolfe HJ, DeLellis RA (1981) Familial medullary carcinoma and C-cell hyperplasia. In: Clinics in Endocrinology and Metabolism, Vol 10/II. Saunders, Eastbourne

Zaloznik AJ, Oswald SG, Longin M (1983) Intrapleural tetracycline in malignant pleural effusions. Cancer 51:752

Zechmann W, Falkensammer M, Wacker H, Jakse G, Zambelis N (1981) Schrittweise Kombination von Skelettszintigramm und Röntgen zur Verbesserung und Rationalisierung des Metastasennachweises im Skelettsystem. Wien klin Wschr 93:261

zum Winkel K (1975) Die externe Strahlenbehandlung der Struma maligna. Verh Dtsch Ges Inn Med 70:879

Subject Index

MIX
Papier aus verantwortungsvollen Quellen
Paper from responsible sources
FSC® C105338

If you have any concerns about our products,
you can contact us on
ProductSafety@springernature.com

In case Publisher is established outside the EU,
the EU authorized representative is:
Springer Nature Customer Service Center GmbH
Europaplatz 3, 69115 Heidelberg, Germany

Printed by Libri Plureos GmbH
in Hamburg, Germany